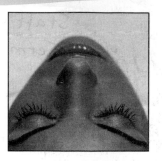

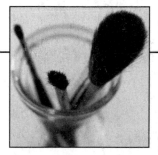

In association with

City & Guilds

BEAUTY THERAPY STUDY SKILLS

NANCY KIRK

me

administrator

Hodder & Stoughton

A MEMBER OF THE HODDER HEADLINE GROUP

This book is dedicated to my husband Edmund,
and my children Rebecca and Cameron

Orders: please contact Bookpoint Ltd, 130 Milton Park, Abingdon, Oxon OX14 4SB.
Telephone: (44) 01235 827720, Fax: (44) 01235 400454. Lines are open from 9.00 – 6.00,
Monday to Saturday, with a 24 hour message answering service. Email address: orders@bookpoint.co.uk

British Library Cataloguing in Publication Data
A catalogue record for this title is available from The British Library

ISBN 0 340 802294

Cover photographs courtesy of Photodisc and DigitalVision.

Typeset by Dorchester Typesetting Ltd
Printed in Great Britain for Hodder & Stoughton Educational, a division of Hodder Headline Plc, 338
Euston Road, London NW1 3BH by Martins The Printers, Berwick Upon Tweed.

ii

CONTENTS

ACKNOWLEDGEMENTS

My special thanks and appreciation must be given to Karen Whitehouse, whose dedication and information technology skills helped bring the original text to life.

Special thanks go to my husband for his endless patience, practical support and encouragement, which has been constant throughout the preparation of this book.

I am especially indebted to Rebecca Morgan for her invaluable advice and checking of the manuscript, and her unfailing encouragement.

Last but not least, I would like to thank Alexandra Lamplugh for her help with many of the diagrams; and also friends and former colleagues from the Beauty Therapy section at Dudley College of Technology, who agreed there was a need for a book around study skills and encouraged me to write it.

My best wishes and thanks to you all.

Nancy Kirk

ABOUT THE AUTHOR

Nancy Kirk has extensive experience in the field of beauty therapy, both as a practitioner and external examiner. She has lectured at all levels of the subject for over two decades, and throughout this time has acted as an external examiner and verifier for the International Health and Beauty Council and City and Guilds. She currently serves as a Subject Specialist Consultant for the City and Guilds of London Institute.

Ever at the forefront of her field, Nancy Kirk is the creator of the City and Guilds Beauty Therapy Progression Award at Level II, and is currently working as a team member for Level III. She also acts as an International Advisor and Educator.

PREFACE

My lengthy experience as a lecturer and external examiner identified a gap for a book such as *Beauty Therapy Study Skills*. I found that students, especially the mature or returning students, needed a lot of support and preparation for end tests, assessments and examinations, and particularly practice in answering examination questions. Furthermore, the current trend of reducing teaching hours in further education and training centres has increased the need for such support and preparation.

This book is therefore designed as a tool for any student undertaking any award in beauty therapy at level II, to overcome these problems. The book is divided into eight succinct chapters, each of which contains a checklist or aide memoir to focus the student on the knowledge they should have when facing end tests or examinations. There are extensive guidelines as to what is likely to be assessed, thus encouraging students to focus their revision on the most relevant points. In each chapter there are simple Revision Maps and sample questions and answers in both multiple choice and short answer style, and some helpful tips to improve answering techniques. Each chapter ends with an end test, and Chapter 8 concludes with a final multiple choice question paper covering all areas of this book.

Throughout this book, the idea is to expose the student to the many styles of testing that they may have to face, thus providing practice and building confidence. New approaches have been used in the form of scenarios, hopefully encouraging the student to think more laterally, and develop deeper understanding of the subject matter. The Revision Maps will also be useful for students with poor organisational skills as they can be used to replace revision notes, and they have the extra benefit of being illustrative as well as textual.

Nancy Kirk

HEALTH, SAFETY AND HYGIENE FOR THE BEAUTY SALON

CHECKLIST ✓ Can You?

HEALTH, SAFETY AND HYGIENE

Hygiene practices and health and safety regulations are observed and assessed continually in the practical situation. People's knowledge of the Health and Safety at Work Act 1974 is often a little confused, and doesn't get any clearer until something unfortunate like an accident occurs. Obviously this is the worst way to learn about health and safety.

This chapter aims to help you understand and revise the various Acts and Regulations that apply to beauty therapists at work. There is also a section to assist your revision and understanding around salon hygiene and the spreading of infection and disease.

The overall aim of the chapter is to 'bring home' the main points that you should know. By no means does the chapter content provide an exhaustive and complete text based on the principles of the Health and Safety at Work Act, but it does provide the relevant material, in an easy-to-understand format. In examinations and tests there will always be *some* questions around health, safety and hygiene. These areas are tested because beauty therapists have a responsibility to the public, and the performance of beauty treatments and the salon environment must always be as safe and hygienic as possible.

Revision Maps are provided around the main areas applicable to the beauty salon and its staff. These are followed by short answer questions and answers, and examples of health and safety scenarios with questions and answers. There is also a short multiple choice test for you to complete (along with answers), and a final end test completes the chapter.

HEALTH AND SAFETY ACTS AND REGULATIONS

Because there are quite a number of different Acts and Regulations, this topic has been divided over four revision maps: Maps A, B, C, D.

When revising, try to learn 'a map at a time', and don't move on to the next map until you are sure you know the information on the map you are studying.

Revision Map – The Health and Safety at Work Act 1974

This Act is very important and should be incorporated into every aspect of the business

The Health and Safety at Work Act 1974

Sometimes called the Umbrella Act, as a lot of regulations are encompassed in it. This Act covers all aspects of Health, Safety and Welfare at work.

The Health and Safety at Work Act is there to protect employees and also the employer.

It clearly states both employer, and employee duties required to safeguard the health, safety and welfare of all.

Main Employer Duties
- Provide and maintain a safe and healthy place of work.
- Ensure effective health and safety policies are in place.
- Provide training and supervision to ensure health and safety procedures are observed and understood.

So, what could happen if the Health and Safety at Work Act is not adhered to and an accident occurs?
- A claim against the business could be made by staff or clients.
- Prosecution and a fine could be the result.
- The business reputation could be severely damaged: *"Clients have long memories"*.

Main Employee Duties
- Cooperate with the employer and observe the salon health and safety procedures.
- Be responsible for the health and safety of the public, colleagues and themselves.

So, who is the Health and Safety Executive?
- A Government body set up to help and advise people about health and safety issues.

So, who are Environmental Health Officers?
- People who work for the Health and Safety Executive.
- They check on standards.
- If they are not happy, they can issue an improvement notice, normally 21 days, to put things right;
OR
- A prohibition notice can be issued which means the salon closes until things are put right.

Revision Map – Control of the Salon Environment

Remember!
Careful control of the salon environment protects the operator and client.

Control of the Salon Environment

Waste Disposal
- Always use a bin with a lid.
- Use a sharps box for contaminated probes or needles.
- All waste bins must be emptied at least once a day. Waste bags should be sealed.
- Any broken glass should be removed with care: use a dustpan and brush, wrap broken glass in several layers of newspaper and label it 'Broken Glass'.

Water Supply
- Clean, fresh hot and cold water is required.
- Don't wash 'solid' materials down the sink (eg Paraffin Wax, Depilatory Wax, lumpy clay mask ingredients), as they could block the sink.
- If a sink becomes blocked, don't leave it. Bad smells and bacterial growth could occur. Report it to your supervisor.

Ventilation
- Very important: fresh air supply crucial to maintaining salon freshness and removes carbon dioxide (CO_2).
- Very important to have an air supply that removes salon smells, eg waxing or manicure smells.
- Keep windows clean.
- Use fans or an air conditioning system if the salon has no windows or restricted air supply.

Maintaining Salon Cleanliness
- Always keep the salon tidy.
- Follow the salon cleaning rota.
- Use appropriate products to clean different items.
- Always tidy up between clients.

Salon which is too hot could result in:
- Uncomfortable clients and staff.
- Fainting occurrences.
- Panic attack occurrences.
- Breathing problems for people with bronchial conditions.

Make sure you know how to control the temperature thermostat.
Make sure you know how to open the windows.

Lighting
- Natural daylight is the most desirable light to have.
- Lighting must be bright enough to allow the operator to see what they are doing. This includes working in stock rooms or storage areas.
- Lighting should be bright enough to allow persons to move around freely.
- Areas like stairs and cloakrooms must be well lit.
- Change flickering or glaring lights immediately.
- Good lighting minimises operator eye strain.

Heating
Working temperature should be 16°C after the first hour.

Micro-Organisms
These multiply more rapidly at around 22°C, so try to maintain a cooler salon.

Revision Map – Beauty Products and Control of Substances Hazardous to Health

COSHH

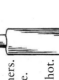

Hydrogen Peroxide
Irritant to the skin and eyes.
- Wear gloves when handling.
- Store in a cool, dry place.
- Never store with combustible material.

Some sterilising agents, equipment cleanser, eyelash tint, nail glue, most artificial nail products
Sensitising – risk of skin reactions.
- Store in a cool, cry place.
- Handle with care.
- Wear gloves if appropriate.

Skin Bleach
Irritating to the skin.
- Wear gloves for handling.
- Avoid inhalation or contact with the eyes.
- Store in a cool, dry place.

Aerosols, eg nail drying spray
Flammable, pressurised containers.
- Keep away from naked flame.
- Don't inhale.
- Don't allow cans to become hot.

Gluteraldehyde Solution
Irritant
- Risk of allergic reactions to the vapour.
- Wear gloves for handling, avoid skin contact.
- Store in a cool, dry place.

Fine Powders, Clay Mask Powders, Talcum Powder, Acrylic Nail Powder, Bleaches
Irritation occurs if you breathe in the particles.
- Don't breathe these products in when mixing them.
- Wear a face mask if necessary.
- Store in a cool, dry place.

Acetone products, Thinners, Surgical Spirit, Witch-hazel, some sterilising agents
Flammable
- Don't smoke when handling these materials.
- Don't breathe in vapours; ensure adequate ventilation when using these products.
- Store in a cool, dry place; don't store large quantities together.
- To dispose of large quantities, contact Environmental Health.

What if there's a problem?
- If reaction occurs on the skin or eyes, rinse freely for 15 minutes.
- If problems occur through inhalation, step into the fresh air. Seek medical advice if you feel no better within 15 minutes, or breathing becomes difficult.

Cuticle Remover
Caustic – can burn.
- Avoid contact with eyes.
- Wear gloves to mop up spillages.
- Store in a cool, dry place.

IRRITANT

INFLAMMABLE LIQUID

Revision Map A

- COSHH   or   Control of Substances Hazardous to Health Act 1989
- RIDDOR or   Reporting of Injuries, Diseases and Dangerous Occurrences Regulations 1985
- PPE   or   Personal Protective Equipment at Work Regulations 1992.

Revision Map B

- The Electricity at Work Regulations 1990
- The Fire Precautions Act 1971
- The Provision and Use of Work Equipment Regulations 1992.

Revision Map C

- The Environmental Protection Act 1990
- The Health and Safety (Display Screen Equipment) Regulations 1992
- The Workplace (Health, Safety and Welfare) Regulations 1992.

Revision Map D

- The Manual Handling Operations Regulations 1992
- The Local Government (Miscellaneous Provisions) Act 1982
- The Management of Health and Safety at Work Regulations 1992.

These are followed by another set of Revision Maps which focus on hygiene and the prevention of infection in the beauty salon.

Revision Map A –
Health and Safety Acts and Regulations

Control of Substances Hazardous to Health Act 1989
COSHH
- Employers must train staff so that they know any risks that are associated with the products used in the workplace, ie Beauty Salon.
- Employers should devise strict rules and procedures for handling, storing, using and disposing of hazardous substances.

The Reporting of Injuries, Diseases and Dangerous Occurrences Regulations 1985
RIDDOR
- All occurrences and incidents should be documented in the salon Accident Book.
- Information regarding injury or incidents at work is passed on to the employer and, if necessary, to the local enforcing authority.

Health and Safety Acts and Regulations
MAP A

So protective equipment for beauty therapy would include:
- Waxing apron and gloves.
- Rubber gloves for handling chemicals like sterilising fluids and equipment cleaner.
- Face masks for handling fine powders or strong chemicals.

The Personal Protective Equipment at Work Regulations 1992
PPE
Employers must provide protective equipment to any employees who may be exposed to health risks or injury.

DANGER
HAZARDOUS MATERIAL STORAGE AREA

Remember, these type of products are all stored in a cool, dry place away from sunlight. These products can affect the skin, the eyes or the lungs through inhalation.

Revision Map B –
Health and Safety Acts and Regulations

The Electricity at Work Regulations 1990
- Electrical appliances/equipment to be tested at least once a year by a qualified electrician.
- Testing must be *properly recorded*.
- Electrical appliances/equipment must be maintained properly and in good working order.

The Fire Precautions Act 1971
- All staff must be trained in fire and emergency evacuation procedures.
- All premises should have adequate means of escape in the case of fire.

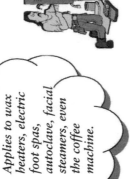

Applies to wax heaters, electric foot spas, autoclave, facial steamers, even the coffee machine.

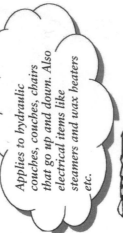

Applies to hydraulic couches, couches, chairs that go up and down. Also electrical items like steamers and wax heaters etc.

Health and Safety Acts and Regulations

MAP B

You should know where fire fighting equipment is located and what extinguisher is to be used on the different types of fire.

You should know
- Where the fire exits are.
- You must never obstruct exits.
Also
- Favourite items in the Beauty Salon for catching fire are wax units and nail products and; favourite causes are clients and therapists who smoke.

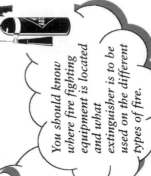

The Provision and use of Work Equipment Regulations 1992
- Equipment used in the salon must be suitable for its purpose.
- All staff must be trained in the correct use of equipment.
- These regulations also apply to second-hand equipment.
- All maintenance to be properly recorded.

Revision Map C –
Health and Safety Acts and Regulations

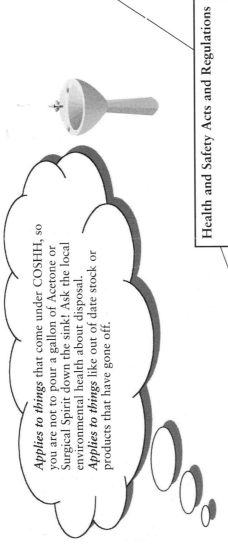

Applies to things that come under COSHH, so you are not to pour a gallon of Acetone or Surgical Spirit down the sink! Ask the local environmental health about disposal.
Applies to things like out of date stock or products that have gone off.

Health and Safety Acts and Regulations

MAP C

The Environmental Protection Act 1990
- The disposal of hazardous substances must not cause harm to anyone or the environment.
- Chemicals must be disposed of safely.

The Health and Safety (Display Screen Equipment) Regulations 1992
- Employers must assess the risks to their employees if they use a VDU (Visual Display Unit) most of the time they are at work.
- Identified risks must be dealt with, eg provide a properly designed chair, eliminate glare by fitting blinds.

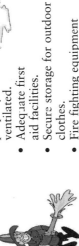

The Workplace (Health, Safety and Welfare) Regulations 1992
- Provides strict regulations about the working environment and employee welfare. *Some* examples include

- Floors, passages, stairs to be free of debris.
- Dust and fumes controlled.
- Sufficient number of toilets, kept clean and properly ventilated.
- Adequate first aid facilities.
- Secure storage for outdoor clothes.
- Fire fighting equipment available.
- Secure fixtures and fittings, etc, etc.

These regulations were brought in to update the 1963 Railway Shops and Premises Act in relation to business premises and safety facilities.

Revision Map D –
Health and Safety Acts and Regulations

The Manual Handling Operations Regulations 1992
- Employers should assess the *risks* in manual handling of loads.
- Training should be provided so staff know how to lift and handle safely.
- Equipment should be provided, eg trolleys, if assessed to be needed.
- Employees should cooperate with employers, take reasonable care when lifting, and use lifting equipment if it's available.

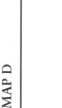

Health and Safety Acts and Regulations

MAP D

The Local Government (Miscellaneous Provisions) Act 1982
- Persons who carry out treatments like ear piercing, electrolysis or micro-pigmentation must be registered with the Local Authority.
- Salons must also be registered and meet certain standards to obtain registration (hygiene, etc).

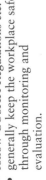

The Management of Health and Safety at Work Regulations 1992
The employer must:
- manage the health and safety process.
- carry out risk assessments.
- record all findings properly.
- provide health and safety training.
- display the poster 'Health and Safety Law'.
- keep all equipment in appropriate order and up to standard.
- consult with staff about health and safety matters.
- follow COSHH Regulations etc.
- generally keep the workplace safe through monitoring and evaluation.

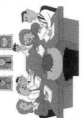

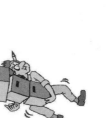

Remember!
Many lifting injuries are caused over a period of time, back injuries, sprains and strains are the most common.
Always take care when lifting stock or moving equipment.

Revision Map – Spreading of Infection and Disease

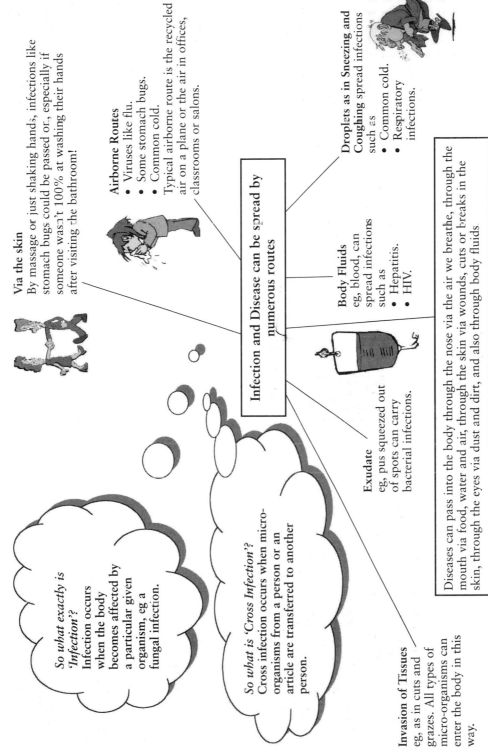

Via the skin
By massage or just shaking hands, infections like stomach bugs could be passed or, especially if someone wasn't 100% at washing their hands after visiting the bathroom!

Airborne Routes
- Viruses like flu.
- Some stomach bugs.
- Common cold.

Typical airborne route is the recycled air on a plane or the air in offices, classrooms or salons.

Droplets as in Sneezing and Coughing spread infections such as
- Common cold.
- Respiratory infections.

Infection and Disease can be spread by numerous routes

Body Fluids
eg, blood, can spread infections such as
- Hepatitis.
- HIV.

Exudate
eg, pus squeezed out of spots can carry bacterial infections.

So what exactly is 'Infection'?
Infection occurs when the body becomes affected by a particular given organism, eg a fungal infection.

So what is 'Cross Infection'?
Cross infection occurs when micro-organisms from a person or an article are transferred to another person.

Invasion of Tissues
eg, as in cuts and grazes. All types of micro-organisms can enter the body in this way.

Diseases can pass into the body through the nose via the air we breathe, through the mouth via food, water and air, through the skin via wounds, cuts or breaks in the skin, through the eyes via dust and dirt, and also through body fluids

Revision Map – Micro-Organisms

Micro-Organisms

Fungi
- Are parasites.
- They live off a host cell, examples include:
  - *Tinea pedis* – **athlete's foot**
    This is a micro-organism that lives in your skin cells. It's a fungi-type micro-organism.
  - *Onycomycosis* – **fungal infection of the nail**
    This is where the micro-organism lives in the nail cells; it's also a fungi-type micro-organism.
- Fungi can multiply by themselves.

An Interesting Fact!
80% of the population will suffer with athlete's foot. There are more cases in men than women.

Viruses
- Are the most resistant micro-organisms.
- They are very difficult to destroy because they enter the *nucleus* of the *host cell*.
- Viruses live within the host cell, and every time the cell multiplies, so does the virus.
- Viruses are not able to multiply by themselves.
- So when the virus is floating in the air as a particle it is harmless. When it makes contact with the body we have a problem.

Examples of viruses include
- Verruca plantaris (verruca on the bottom surface of the foot), measles, hepatitis, mumps, rabies, herpes simplex.

Bacteria
- Typically consist of a single cell that has a protective wall.
- Some bacteria need oxygen and infect areas like the skin or lungs, eg impetigo, pneumonia.
- Some bacteria can exist in oxygen-free areas, eg in the bowel or stomach.
- Bacteria can release toxins that harm body cells or can produce an inflammatory response.
- Bacteria can multiply by themselves.
- Bacteria can cause horrible diseases like salmonella, meningitis, whooping cough.
- Bacteria can be very resilient.
- Not all bacteria cause disease, some are helpful to man.
- Bacteria can live on tools and equipment, in pedicure bowls, on salon surfaces, trolleys and couches and lots of other places.

Revision Map – Terminology of Salon Hygiene

Terminology of Salon Hygiene

Sterilising
The process used to render equipment or articles free of all micro-organisms and their spores.

Sterile
Free from all micro-organisms and their spores.

Sanitisation
The procedures carried out to prevent the spread of disease.

Cut Out System
The way in which professional therapists transfer products from containers for use on clients. Spatulae are always used. A spatula that has touched the skin is never re-entered into the product.

Disinfection is used to render objects, room surfaces, and even people from harmful micro-organisms. *Think!* We disinfect treatment couches, manicure bowls, manicure and make-up trays, walls and floors.

A **Disinfectant** is a toxic chemical that will kill *most* micro-organisms, making the disinfected environment safer. Examples include:

Gluteraldehyde – a 2% strength is used. (Irritant COSHH). Can be used to soak metal instruments and applicators. Can stain the skin brown so work with care during handling. Can use on blood spillages.

Hypochlorites – Common bleaches contain calcium or sodium hypochlorite. These are very inexpensive so good for general cleaning and soaking plastics. Irritant COSHH so use with care. Corrosive to some tools and equipment.

Alcohols, 70% alcohol content eg Surgical Spirit can be used on the skin, perhaps in wiping over the feet prior to body massage.
eg Methylated Spirit – ideal for wiping over mirrors and tiled surfaces.

Antiseptics
- Substances used to limit and prevent the growth of micro-organisms.
- Can be used on the skin.
- Proper antiseptics are chemicals, so use with care.
- Many brand name antiseptic solutions and products are available.
- Therapists should use an antiseptic to wash hands prior to treatment.
- Therapists should use an antiseptic to wipe over the hands, feet and waxing areas.

Remember! Some products used in the sanitisation and disinfection processes need to be diluted. Always dilute properly.
Remember! Certain disinfectant products like gluteraldehyde need time to work and lose their effectiveness after a period of time. Always follow manufacturer guidelines.
Gluteraldehydes are commonly used for soaking tools and equipment.

Revision Map – Different Methods of Sterilisation commonly used in the Beauty Salon

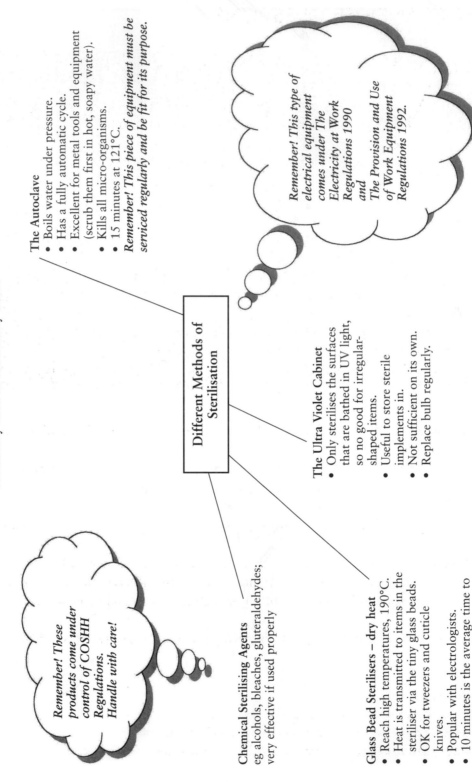

Different Methods of Sterilisation

The Autoclave
- Boils water under pressure.
- Has a fully automatic cycle.
- Excellent for metal tools and equipment (scrub them first in hot, soapy water).
- Kills all micro-organisms.
- 15 minutes at 121°C.
Remember! This piece of equipment must be serviced regularly and be fit for its purpose.

Remember! This type of electrical equipment comes under The Electricity at Work Regulations 1990 and The Provision and Use of Work Equipment Regulations 1992.

The Ultra Violet Cabinet
- Only sterilises the surfaces that are bathed in UV light, so no good for irregular-shaped items.
- Useful to store sterile implements in.
- Not sufficient on its own.
- Replace bulb regularly.

Chemical Sterilising Agents
eg alcohols, bleaches, gluteraldehydes; very effective if used properly

Remember! These products come under control of COSHH Regulations. Handle with care!

Glass Bead Sterilisers – dry heat
- Reach high temperatures, 190°C.
- Heat is transmitted to items in the steriliser via the tiny glass beads.
- OK for tweezers and cuticle knives.
- Popular with electrologists.
- 10 minutes is the average time to have desired effect.

SHORT ANSWER QUESTIONS

 REMEMBER!

1. Read through each question carefully.
2. Look at how many marks are awarded for each question.

3. **Think** How would I answer this question to gain the maximum marks available.
4. Read through the answer provided.
5. **Ask yourself:**
   Was the answer clear?
   Did it answer the question?
   Would this answer attract full marks from the marker?
   Did the answer include any unnecessary waffle?
   Always:
   Avoid writing unnecessary waffle when answering questions.
   Examiners hate marking it.
   Answer the question clearly and fully, but no more and nothing less.

Q1. Under COSHH regulations, what does the term 'Irritant' mean? *(2 marks)*

Answer: In this situation, the word irritant denotes that a product or substance could have an adverse effect on the skin or the organs of respiration.

Q2. How should 'Irritant' products be labelled? *(3 marks)*

Answer: Standard symbols are used to classify hazardous substances. The symbol for irritant is a large letter X. Ideally the name of the product should also be stated, eg Hydrogen Peroxide. All labels must be big enough to be seen and easily read.

Q3. Give two examples of beauty therapy products that are flammable.

(2 marks)

Answer:
- Aerosols, eg nail drying sprays, foot powders.
- Acetone products, eg nail enamel remover, nail enamel solvent.
- Other possible answers include surgical spirit, astringent, witch-hazel.

Q4. What is the role of the Health and Safety Executive? *(5 marks)*

Answer: The Health and Safety Executive is the leading Government Body which provides material, help and advice on issues regarding health and safety in the workplace. The Health and Safety Executive has a series of offices set up throughout the country from which these activities take place. It is able to enforce health and safety regulations, and in circumstances where the health and safety law has been broken, it has the power to prevent a business from trading, or to issue 'improvement notices' (detailing how improvements must be made, together with a time limit by which the improvements must be implemented).

Q5. How does the Local Government (Miscellaneous Provisions) Act 1982 affect salons that carry out ear-piercing? *(3 marks)*

Answer: This Act requires all persons who perform ear-piercing to be registered with the Local Authority. The salon must also be registered and will have to meet certain criteria to obtain registration. The criteria is aimed to maintain acceptable standards of cleanliness, hygiene and sterilisation.

Q6. State how diseases can be passed into the body. *(6 marks)*

Answer: Diseases can be passed into the body via a number of routes;
• Through the nose in the air we breathe.
• Through the mouth by food and water and the air we breathe.
• Through the skin via breaks or wounds in the skin.
• Through the eyes when dust and dirt enter them.
Diseases, bacteria and viruses can also be spread via body fluid contact.

Q7. Give two examples of infections caused through droplets. *(2 marks)*

Answer:
1. The common cold.
2. Respiratory infections.

Q8. Name two conditions that can be passed on through contact with contaminated body fluid. *(2 marks)*

Answer:
1. HIV.
2. Hepatitis.

Q9. How do the micro-organisms fungi and bacteria differ from viruses?

(3 marks)

Answer: Fungi and bacteria are able to multiply by themselves. Viruses are not able to complete this function; they multiply as and when the host cell, within which they exist, multiplies.

Q10. How should lighting be maintained in a stockroom where there is no natural light?

(5 marks)

Answer: Any bulbs or fluorescent tubes which have blown must be replaced immediately. Any shades or coverings on lights must be kept clean. Ideally, lighting should be positioned to provide illumination where it is needed, eg on aisles, and in areas where people can see what they are doing without losing the light source to the top of shelving or racking.

Q11. Name four items of tools and equipment which are used for unpacking stock which could be dangerous if not used properly.

(4 marks)

Answer: Any four from this list: scissors, knives or blades, staple removers, claw hammers, crow bars.

Q12. Why are fine powders like fuller's earth and talcum powder included in COSHH Regulations?

(2 marks)

Answer: Because they are products that could be irritating if they are inhaled.

Q13. Why could hydrogen peroxide be a 'health hazard', and how must this product be stored?

(4 marks)

Answer: Hydrogen peroxide can be hazardous if it is in contact with the skin or the eyes because it is an irritant. It must be stored in a cool dry place, away from other combustible products.

Q14. Briefly outline the main employee duties required by the Health and Safety at Work Act 1974.

(4 marks)

Answer: The employee must cooperate with the employer in their efforts to provide a safe and healthy place of work. Employees must be responsible for the health and safety of the public, colleagues and themselves.

Q15. What *Regulations* state that 'Staff must be trained in the correct use of equipment'? *(1 mark)*

Answer: The Provision and Use of Work Equipment Regulations 1992.

Q16. What must the beauty therapist do to uphold the Fire Precautions Act 1971? Give three examples *(6 marks)*

Answer:
1. Ensure that they undergo training in salon evacuation and fire procedures, and know where the fire exits are.
2. Be aware of the location of fire-fighting equipment and know the correct use of it.
3. Ensure that exits, passages and corridors are never obstructed.

Q17. Give an example of how the Electricity at Work Regulations 1990 apply to beauty therapy equipment. *(4 marks)*

Answer: Under these regulations all electrical appliances/equipment must be tested by a *qualified* electrician at *least once a year*. The testing procedure must be properly recorded. This means that all salon electrical equipment, eg wax units, facial steamers, sterilisers, electrical foot spas, etc, must undergo this inspection to comply with these regulations.

Q18. Explain why the Health and Safety at Work Act 1974 is sometimes called 'The Encompassing Act' or 'The Umbrella Act'. *(6 marks)*

Answer: In general terms, Acts like the Health and Safety at Work Act 1974 set out the main *points* and *objectives* to be achieved. Regulations are much more clearly written, and are often incorporated into the appropriate Act months or years later. This happened in 1992, when six new sets of more strict regulations about health and safety were introduced, following directives from the European Union. These new regulations were all incorporated into the Health and Safety at Work Act.
Student Note! An example of the new regulations is the Health and Safety (Display Screen Equipment) Regulations 1992.

Q19. Give two examples of how the Personal Protective Equipment at Work Regulations 1992 could apply to a beauty therapist in the carrying-out of salon duties. *(5 marks)*

Answer: These regulations state that employers must provide protective equipment to any employees who may be exposed to health risks or injury.

1. Some employers may provide surgical gloves for depilatory waxing and request that they are worn by the therapist during waxing treatments. If this is part of the salon's health and safety policy, it must be adhered to.

2. If employers provide face masks and/or rubber gloves for staff to wear during cleaning or dispensing of stock, they should also be used appropriately.

Q20. Why does having adequate ventilation contribute to a healthier salon environment? *(2 marks)*

Answer: Adequate ventilation is important because it helps to maintain the fresh air supply of the salon, thus maintaining salon freshness and the removal of carbon dioxide and smells generated by salon treatments.

Q21. Why do many salon basins include an 'S' bend as part of their plumbing? *(3 marks)*

Answer: The 'S' bend acts as a waste trap and catches any small objects that could have fallen through the plug hole. Also the 'S' bend is effective in preventing unpleasant smells or gasses travelling back up through the pipes.

Q22. What is an antiseptic and when might one be used in an underarm waxing treatment? *(5 marks)*

Answer: An antiseptic is a substance (normally chemical) which is used on the skin to limit and prevent the growth of micro-organisms. In an underarm waxing treatment, an antiseptic would be used prior to treatment as part of the preparation process, and also on completion, where it would probably be applied as an antiseptic soothing cream or lotion.

Q23. Give an example of a suitable product for general disinfection of mirrored and glass surfaces. *(1 mark)*

Answer: Methylated spirit.

Q24. What percentage alcohol is present in the product known as Surgical Spirit? *(1 mark)*

Answer: 70%.

Q25. Explain the meaning of the term 'sterile'   *(2 marks)*

Answer: 'Sterile' is used to describe a state where an object or item, or even an atmosphere, is free from all micro-organisms and their spores.

Q26. If a spillage of nail enamel remover was on fire, what fire extinguisher should *not* be used?   *(1 mark)*

Answer: The *Red* fire extinguisher.

Q27. When might a bucket of sand be used to fight a fire?   *(1 mark)*

Answer: Sand can be used to smother a fire and is especially useful to extinguish small fires caused by flammable liquids.

Q28. Under what circumstances would you use the *Black, Carbon Dioxide* fire extinguisher?   *(2 marks)*

Answer: The *black* extinguisher is safe for use on all electrical fires and flammable liquids.

HEALTH AND SAFETY SCENARIOS

The following health and safety scenarios, questions and answers enable you to see how everyday salon activities could lead to health and safety legislation being broken. Reading through the questions and answers will enable you to experience different styles of questioning, and expose you to acceptable answering techniques.

Look through the following text and then review the example questions and answers. All questions and answers are based on the information given as Example One.

Example One

Jane has a very busy salon; she employs two therapists and works full-time in the business. Jane has been in business for two years and has had a general electrical service and testing 14 months ago. She has just found some old stock that belonged to the previous owners and has instructed the junior therapist to pour it down the sink. The old stock contains gallons of eau de cologne, surgical spirit, cleansers, rancid almond oil and a gluteraldehyde solution. The junior therapist has just informed Jane that the supply of surgical gloves has just ran out, and there are four ear-piercing clients booked later on that afternoon.

Q1. With regard to the electrical equipment, which regulations are being broken?

Answer: The Electricity at Work Regulations 1990 are not being adhered to. These regulations state that electrical appliances/equipment *must* be tested at least once a year by a qualified electrician. As the last service and check was 14 months ago, this is unacceptable. Also, the Provision of Work Equipment Regulations 1992 are being breached. These regulations state that all equipment must be suitable and fit for its purpose. As no testing has taken place for some 14 months it cannot be deemed that equipment is truly fit for its purpose.

Q2. The junior therapist has been instructed to pour 'gallons' of old stock down the sink.
a) Why could the disposal of these products in this way be undesirable?
b) Ideally, what action should the employer have taken to ensure safe disposal of these products.

Answer:
a) The disposal of some of these products could have broken the Environmental Protection Act 1990. This Act states that *chemicals* must be disposed of safely. Surgical spirit and gluteraldehyde are chemicals, and in this quantity they could be problematical to the environment. Also, eau de cologne is flammable and is generally handled according to the COSHH regulations.
b) The employer should contact the Environmental Health Department who will provide advice about the disposal of these products. The employer may be directed to take the products to a certain disposal point, or retain them for collection and disposal by the Environmental Health Department.

Q3. This salon carries out ear-piercing treatments.
a) What legislation governs this type of treatment?
b) Is it advisable to perform ear-piercing treatments without gloves? Justify your answer.

Answer:

a) Any premises that carries out ear-piercing treatments must be registered with their local authority. This is a requirement of the Local Government (Miscellaneous Provisions) Act 1982.

b) It is not advisable to perform this treatment without gloves because there is the risk of blood appearing at the site of the piercing; body fluids such as blood can carry the HIV virus and the hepatitis virus. Also, performing this treatment without gloves would be in contravention of local government regulations which could lead to registration being withdrawn.

Example two

'Beauty One' is a large health and beauty centre employing 25 full-time staff. A large delivery has just arrived containing 30 boxes of beauty and health products. The technician who received the order has requested the help of the junior therapist and the second receptionist to move the stock which is blocking the fire exit. The technician is the only person of the three who has been trained in manual handling operations. A cage has been sent for, to carry the stock to the storeroom. When the cage arrives, the junior begins to stack the cage with no regard to the size or content of the boxes. The technician intervenes and re-arranges the packages in a productive manner. The cage is fully stacked, its doors are closed, and the fire exit is now clear. The technician is diverted by a client, and the junior and second receptionist begin to drag the cage in the direction of the storeroom.

Q1. Who is responsible for assessing the risks in the manual handling of loads?

Answer: The employer is responsible for conducting this type of risk assessment.

Q2. The stock was blocking a fire exit. What action should be taken to avoid this happening again, and which regulations were breached by this occurrence?

Answer: The employer has overall responsibility to ensure that fire exits are never blocked or obstructed in any way. In this scenario, the employer could be criticised under the Management of Health and Safety at Work Regulations 1992 and would need to urgently review the procedures in place for receiving stock. New, safer procedures must be implemented and all relevant staff should receive training. The technician should not have allowed the fire exit to become blocked.

The employer needs to review the health and safety training for the technician so that this type of incident does not occur again. The Fire Precautions Act 1971 was being breached by allowing the fire exit to become blocked.

Q3. Identify three training needs of the junior therapist.

Answer: The junior therapist would benefit from training in manual handling operations. Also there is a strong likelihood that in this delivery of 30 boxes, some of the contents would need to be handled in line with COSHH regulations, and not stacked in the manner described. Training is therefore also needed in COSHH and the rules and procedures for the safe stacking of goods.

Q4. How should a cage (with the doors closed) be transported from place to place?

Answer: A cage or roll pallet should always be pushed, not pulled.

Q5. In this incidence, was it advisable to use a cage with doors to transport the stock? Justify your answer.

Answer: Yes, this is an ideal way to move stock. Clearly the employer would have assessed that this piece of equipment was needed to avoid risk of injury to staff. It is the duty of the employee to co-operate with the employer and make use of any appropriate equipment which is provided for them for the safe handling of stock. In this incidence, it was vitally important that the stock was moved quickly to free the fire exit. The use of a cage enabled the process to be carried out swiftly.

Q6. Give two examples of protective clothing that *ideally* should have been provided for the junior therapist. Give the reasons for your answer.

Answer: A protective overall or apron should have been provided to protect the therapist's salon dress. Not only would this item protect clothing from becoming soiled, but it would also maintain hygiene levels if the same salon dress was to be worn for carrying out treatments later in the day.

Protective gloves should also have been worn, which would protect the hands from cuts and abrasions and from any spillage of the contents which could damage the skin.

Q7. Under the Fire Precautions Act 1971, this establishment would be required to have a fire certificate. Why is this?

Answer: Because there are more than 20 personnel employed and working at any one time.

Q8. Which regulations state that employers must provide protective equipment to any employees who may be exposed to health risks or injury?

Answer: The Personal Protective Equipment at Work Regulations 1992.

MULTIPLE CHOICE QUESTIONS

Some examples of multiple choice examination questions are included for you to enable you to give yourself a short test. Carefully consider the descriptions provided before choosing your answer. Only one answer is correct.
Indicate your answer by putting an **X** in the circle. ◯

EXAMPLE QUESTION
The Health and Safety at Work Act became legislation in

a) 1968 ◯

b) 1971 ◯

c) 1974 ⊗

d) 1992 ◯

Correct answer is **c)** 1974

REMEMBER!

1. Carefully read through the test paper.

2. Start by reading the question to yourself twice. Be sure you understand the question.

3. Read the possible answers twice. Use the process of elimination to rule out the incorrect answers. Select your answer.

4. Leave any questions you are unsure of, and come back to them at the end.

5. If faced with any questions you cannot answer, don't be afraid to guess as a last resort.

6. Finally, check through your work, and take your time. Carefully check each question one at a time.

Q1. A general guideline for stacking stock is to:

a) stack heavy stock on top of light stock ○

b) stack stock in tall slender piles ○

c) stack light stock on top of heavy stock ○

d) stack larger items on top of small items ○

Q2. When lifting a low level box of stock, you should:

a) use the muscles in your back keeping your chin up ○

b) use the muscles in your legs ○

c) bend over the load and keep your back straight ○

d) use the muscles in your legs with your back straight and chin in ○

Q3. If a glass bead steriliser is working at a temperature of 190°C, how long would be needed to sterilise a pair of eyebrow tweezers?

a) 10 minutes ○

b) 20 minutes ○

c) 30 minutes ○

d) 60 minutes ○

Q4. The condition known as verruca pedis is caused by:

a) bacteria ○

b) a virus ○

c) a fungi ○

d) poor hygiene ○

Q5. The micro-organism that causes tinea pedis is a:

a) bacteria-type micro-organism ○

b) virus ○

c) fungi-type micro-organism ○

d) super resistant micro-organism ○

Q6. The most resistant micro-organisms are:

a) viruses ◯

b) germs ◯

c) bacteria ◯

d) fungi ◯

Q7. Herpes simplex is caused by:

a) a fungi-type micro-organism ◯

b) harmful bacteria which attack the skin ◯

c) a bacteria-type micro-organism ◯

d) a virus-type micro-organism ◯

Q8. Cages or roll pallets containing stock items should be:

a) pushed with the doors closed ◯

b) pulled with the doors closed ◯

c) pushed along corridors, pulled through doors ◯

d) moved in the most comfortable way possible for the operator, but always with the doors closed ◯

Q9. The hazard symbol or icon that depicts a Skull and Crossbones is used on items that are:

a) corrosive ◯

b) oxidising ◯

c) harmful ◯

d) toxic ◯

Q10. Which *one* of the following items comes under COSHH regulations:

a) calamine lotion ◯

b) magnesium carbonate ◯

c) eye make-up remover ◯

d) anti-bacterial foot soak ◯

Q11. How long does a glass bead steriliser take to reach a temperature capable of sterilising small objects?

a) 10 minutes ○

b) 10–20 minutes ○

c) 30–60 minutes ○

d) 90 minutes ○

Q12. The product gluteraldehyde is used in the salon:

a) during cuticle work in a nail treatment ○

b) during sanitisation procedures ○

c) to prepare the nails prior to enamel application ○

d) for general purpose cleaning ○

Q13. Which one of the following is the best way to prevent and limit the growth of micro-organisms on the skin?

a) wipe over the skin with a 2% gluteraldehyde product ○

b) wipe over the skin with a disinfectant lotion ○

c) wipe over the skin with hot soapy water ○

d) wipe over the skin with an antiseptic substance ○

Q14. The time needed to sterilise items in the autoclave at 121°C is:

a) 3 minutes ○

b) 10 minutes ○

c) 15 minutes ○

d) 20 minutes ○

Q15. An ultra violet cabinet has limited use as a sterilising instrument because:

a) it is very expensive to install ○

b) it only sterilises the surfaces it touches ○

c) the bulbs are difficult to change ○

d) this piece of equipment has links with eye damage and is restricted in use ○

Q16. If a salon is issued with an improvement notice, they have a period in which to improve or put something right. This time period is normally:

a) 7 days ○

b) 21 days ○

c) 28 days ○

d) 30 days ○

Q17. When should a sharps box be used?

a) to dispose of electrolysis needles ○

b) to store electrolysis needles ○

c) to dispose of flammable products ○

d) to dispose of used cotton wool and tissues ○

Q18. Which one of the following is a *sensitising* product controlled by COSHH regulations?

a) surgical spirit ○

b) kaolin ○

c) fuller's earth ○

d) eyelash tint ○

Q19. Which regulations state that incidents and accidents should be documented in the salon accident book?

a) the Personal Protective Equipment at Work Regulations ○

b) the Control of Substances Hazardous to Health Act ○

c) the Reporting of Injuries, Diseases and Dangerous Occurrences regulations ○

d) the Electricity at Work Regulations ○

Q20. The 1963 Railway Shops and Premises Act was updated in 1992 by the introduction of:

a) the Environmental Protection Act ○

b) the Fire Precautions Act ○

c) the Electricity at Work Regulations ○

d) the Workplace (Health, Safety and Welfare) Regulations ○

Q21. Under the Electricity at Work Regulations 1990, who must carry out testing on electrical appliances and equipment?

a) the supervisor ○

b) a qualified electrician ○

c) a qualified engineer ○

d) the manager/manageress ○

Q22. How often should electrical equipment/appliances be tested to comply with regulations? At least:

a) every 6 months ○

b) every 12 months ○

c) every 2 years ○

d) every 3 years ○

Q23. The colour of the fire extinguisher that emits carbon dioxide is:

a) black ○

b) green ○

c) red ○

d) blue ○

Q24. Which fire extinguisher emits water and is used to put out 'paper fires'?

a) green ○

b) black ○

c) cream ○

d) red ○

Q25. Towels and linen which have been in contact with clients should be washed in soapy water at a temperature of:

a) 30°C ○

b) 40°C ○

c) 50°C ○

d) 60°C ○

1.	C	8.	A	15.	B	22.	B
2.	D	9.	D	16.	B	23.	A
3.	A	10.	B	17.	A	24.	D
4.	B	11.	C	18.	D	25.	D
5.	C	12.	B	19.	C		
6.	A	13.	D	20.	D		
7.	D	14.	C	21.	B		

Marking and Grading

20 correct   a credit, excellent

15 correct   a pass, well done

Just below 15   You're nearly there. Keep revising, have a look at the Revision Maps and have another go.

Below 10   You need to spend a bit more time revising. Go back to your course notes and the Revision Maps and have another go in a week's time.

FINAL END TEST

This section consists of statements. Each one may be correct or incorrect. The answer required is simply

Yes or **No.**

In your assessment of whether the statement is correct or incorrect, you must only base your answer on the information provided. After ensuring that all the questions have been answered, check the answers yourself at the end of the chapter.

1. Burning is an effective way to dispose of contaminated waste.

2. An autoclave reaches temperatures above 100°C.

3. Ultra violet cabinets are as effective as autoclaves.

4. A *single* piece of equipment can be sterilised in 10 minutes in a glass bead steriliser.

5. Micro-organisms can enter the body via contaminated foods.

6. Droplet infections cannot be passed on by talking.

7. Viruses are larger than bacterium.

8. All bacteria need oxygen to survive.

9. The temperature of depilatory wax and paraffin wax must be tested on the operator prior to commencing treatment.

10. During hot oil mask treatments there is *no need* to protect the eyes from the rays of the heat lamp.

11. Under the Health and Safety at Work Act 1974, the *employer* is responsible for providing and maintaining a safe and healthy place of work.

12. An 'Improvement Notice' normally gives the recipient 21 days to bring about the required improvement.

13. The salon working temperature should be 16°C after the first hour.

14. Harsh glare from lighting can increase the occurrence of headaches.

15. General salon waste must be disposed of in sealed bags.

〔⎯⎯⎯⎯⎯〕

16. The disinfectant product Gluteraldehyde can be an irritant.

〔⎯⎯⎯⎯⎯〕

17. Under COSHH regulations, talcum powder is classed as flammable.

〔⎯⎯⎯⎯⎯〕

18. A *very serious* incident or accident in the salon would need to be reported as a requirement of RIDDOR.

〔⎯⎯⎯⎯⎯〕

19. Employers are *not* obliged to provide COSHH training.

〔⎯⎯⎯⎯⎯〕

20. Under the Fire Precautions Act 1971, all staff must be trained in fire and emergency evacuation procedures.

〔⎯⎯⎯⎯⎯〕

21. The red fire extinguisher emits water and is suitable for paper, card or wood fires.

〔⎯⎯⎯⎯⎯〕

22. The red fire extinguisher *can* be used on electrical fires.

〔⎯⎯⎯⎯⎯〕

23. Second-hand electrical equipment does not come under the Provision and Use of Work Equipment Regulations 1992.

〔⎯⎯⎯⎯⎯〕

24. The Workplace (Health, Safety and Welfare) Regulations 1992 were brought in to update and improve the Railway Shops and Premises Act and the Health and Safety at Work Act.

〔⎯⎯⎯⎯⎯〕

25. The Local Government (Miscellaneous Provisions) Act 1982 only applies to Tattoo Parlours.

〔⎯⎯⎯⎯⎯〕

26. Micro-organisms can be passed from the skin of an infected person during a massage treatment or simply by shaking a person's hand.

〔⎯⎯⎯⎯⎯〕

27. HIV and Hepatitis are passed on via body fluids.

28. During pedicure treatments gloves can be worn to protect from potential fungal conditions that may be developing.

29. Viruses are fragile micro-organisms.

30. Bacteria can live on tools and equipment, trolleys, work surfaces, brushes and many other objects.

31. The employer is the only person responsible for sanitisation.

32. Antiseptics can be used on the skin.

33. To be classed as a proper disinfectant, surgical spirit should have a 70% alcohol content.

34. Manicure/pedicure tools could be *disinfected* by boiling them rapidly in a pan of boiling water for 10 minutes.

35. The term 'toxic' is used to denote something as being poisonous and able to injure or kill if introduced into a person.

FINAL END TEST **ANSWERS**

1. Yes
2. Yes
3. No   Definitely not. The UV cabinet emits rays that destroy micro-organisms on the surfaces they reach only.
4. Yes
5. Yes
6. No   It is possible to pass on infections in this way also by coughing and sneezing.
7. No   A virus is smaller.
8. No   Some do and some don't. Bacteria that live in the intestines don't have oxygen.
9. Yes
10. No   You should always cover the client's eyes with protective pads prior to application of the lamp.
11. Yes
12. Yes
13. Yes
14. Yes
15. Yes
16. Yes
17. No   Talcum powder is classed as an irritant.
18. Yes
19. No   This is an incorrect statement. Employers must train staff so that they know any risks associated with the products used in the workplace.
20. Yes
21. Yes
22. No   It must never be used on electrical fires. The black CO_2 extinguisher is suitable.
23. No   This is untrue. These regulations apply to all work equipment.
24. Yes

25. No   Untrue. This Act requires salons offering ear-piercing, micro-pigmentation and electrolysis to register their premises and all staff who apply these treatments.

26. Yes

27. Yes

28. Yes

29. No   Untrue. Viruses are the most resistant micro-organisms.

30. Yes

31. No   Sanitisation procedures should be carried out by all employees and the employer to help prevent the spread of disease.

32. Yes

33. Yes

34. Yes   Also this is a good procedure to be included in general hygiene practices and should be carried out weekly.

35. Yes

Marking Guide and Grading

The marking guide is provided to help and encourage you to monitor your progress.

This style of end test has been chosen to reinforce some key revision points to further assist your revision process. Obviously, if you have guessed a lot of the answers, it will not give you a proper reflection of the true mark you have achieved, and really, if you have to guess answers, you need to revise a bit more.

28 correct answers   a credit

25 correct answers   a confident pass

21 correct answers   a borderline pass

Below 21 correct means you need to revise a bit more. Go back to your course notes and Revision Maps, spend some more time studying, and have another go at the test at a later date. Don't be put off, but be prepared to spend some proper time on it.

CHECKLIST ✓ Can You?

	Yes	No	Page No
1. Draw or label a diagram to show the structure of the nail. Describe nail structure and explain the process of nail growth.			38
2. Name and describe the contra-indications that would require the client to be referred to their GP. Name and describe conditions of the nail, hands and feet which can be improved by treatments.			46
3. Write accurately about the tools, ingredients and actions of products that are used in nail treatments.			52
4. Discuss examples of the main bones and muscles of the hand and arm, foot and lower leg.			58
5. Outline the blood circulation to the hands and feet. State the effects of massage on the limbs. State the contra-indications to massage of the limbs.			58
6. Relate methods of maintaining hygiene levels and a safe working environment during treatments.			73
7. Devise treatment plans for clients.			76
8. Attempt a final end test.			88

NAIL STRUCTURE AND GROWTH

The structure of the nail is *always* included in tests and examinations. Knowing about the structure of the nail is the basis for providing nail treatments, and therefore is a favourite questioning point of the examiner. Look at the revision map (page 39) to help focus your revision, and review your course notes. When you feel ready attempt Task 1.

You also need to know how the nail grows, and the factors that can influence the nail growth process. The Revision Map on page 40 should simplify this for you.

TASK 1 Label the diagram below: the structure of the nail

*Helpful Tip! Try not to be put off if the diagram is slightly different to the one you are used to. Take your time. Label first the parts you are sure of, then proceed to the others. Do try and get the spellings correct; it is much more professional.

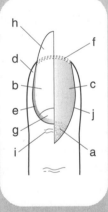

a) Matrix
b) Nail Plate
c) Nail Bed
d) Nail Wall
e) Cuticle or Eponychium
f) Hyponychium
g) Lunula
h) Free Edge
i) Nail Fold or Nail Root
j) Nail Groove

All correct	Excellent
One or two errors	Well done, but go back to the revision map
Many errors	Don't panic. Go back to your course notes and the revision map and then have another go

BEAUTY THERAPY STUDY SKILLS

Revision Map – Nail Structure

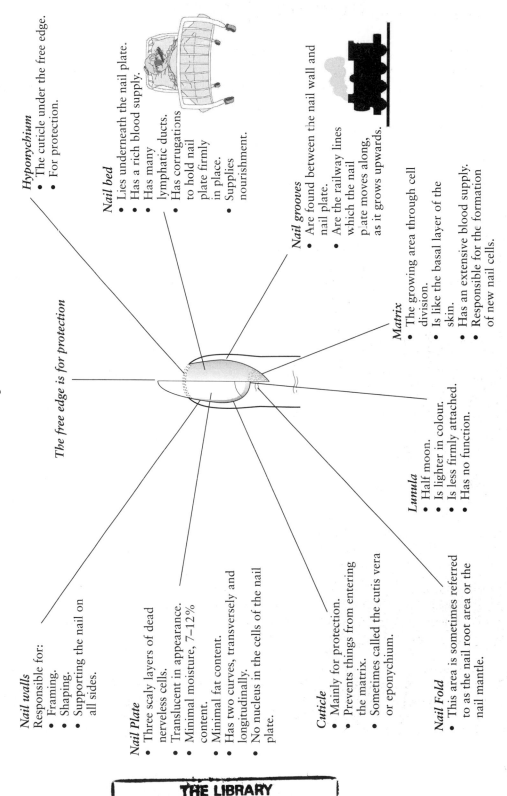

The free edge is for protection

Hyponychium
- The cuticle under the free edge.
- For protection.

Nail bed
- Lies underneath the nail plate.
- Has a rich blood supply.
- Has many lymphatic ducts.
- Has corrugations to hold nail plate firmly in place.
- Supplies nourishment.

Nail grooves
- Are found between the nail wall and nail plate.
- Are the railway lines which the nail plate moves along, as it grows upwards.

Matrix
- The growing area through cell division.
- Is like the basal layer of the skin.
- Has an extensive blood supply.
- Responsible for the formation of new nail cells.

Lunula
- Half moon.
- Is lighter in colour.
- Is less firmly attached.
- Has no function.

Nail walls
Responsible for:
- Framing.
- Shaping.
- Supporting the nail on all sides.

Nail Plate
- Three scaly layers of dead nerveless cells.
- Translucent in appearance.
- Minimal moisture, 7–12% content.
- Minimal fat content.
- Has two curves, transversely and longitudinally.
- No nucleus in the cells of the nail plate.

Cuticle
- Mainly for protection.
- Prevents things from entering the matrix.
- Sometimes called the cutis vera or eponychium.

Nail Fold
- This area is sometimes referred to as the nail root area or the nail mantle.

Revision Map – The Process of Nail Growth

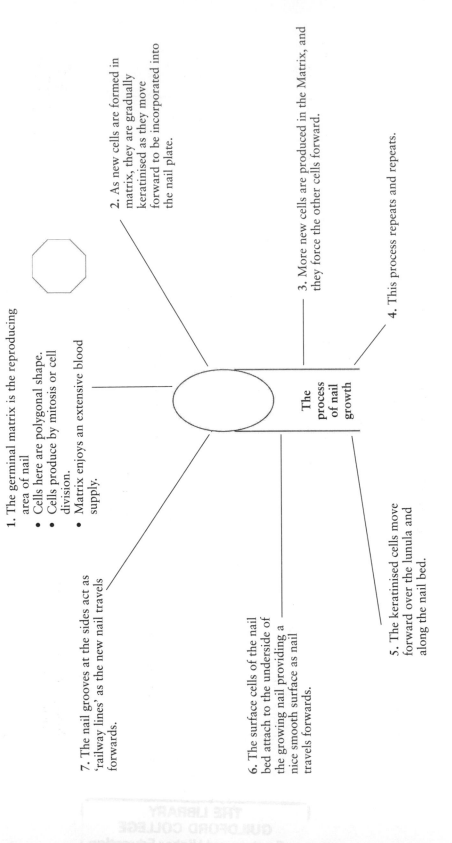

The process of nail growth

1. The germinal matrix is the reproducing area of nail
   - Cells here are polygonal shape.
   - Cells produce by mitosis or cell division.
   - Matrix enjoys an extensive blood supply.

2. As new cells are formed in matrix, they are gradually keratinised as they move forward to be incorporated into the nail plate.

3. More new cells are produced in the Matrix, and they force the other cells forward.

4. This process repeats and repeats.

5. The keratinised cells move forward over the lumula and along the nail bed.

6. The surface cells of the nail bed attach to the underside of the growing nail providing a nice smooth surface as nail travels forwards.

7. The nail grooves at the sides act as 'railway lines' as the new nail travels forwards.

Revision Map – General Facts about Nail Growth

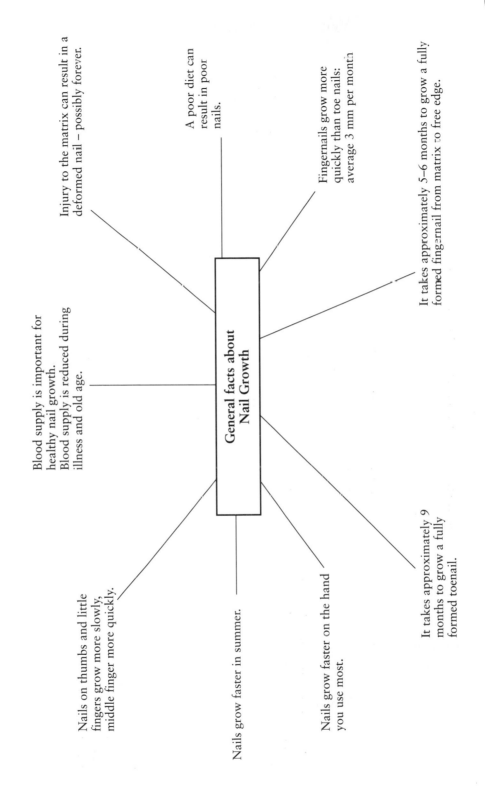

General facts about Nail Growth

Injury to the matrix can result in a deformed nail – possibly forever.

A poor diet can result in poor nails.

Fingernails grow more quickly than toe nails: average 3 mm per month.

It takes approximately 5–6 months to grow a fully formed fingernail from matrix to free edge.

Blood supply is important for healthy nail growth. Blood supply is reduced during illness and old age.

Nails on thumbs and little fingers grow more slowly, middle finger more quickly.

Nails grow faster in summer.

Nails grow faster on the hand you use most.

It takes approximately 9 months to grow a fully formed toenail.

SHORT ANSWER QUESTIONS

An example of some model questions and answers are provided to help give you an insight on how to answer questions properly. Reading through the questions and answers will also help your revision.

Question: Describe the position and function of the matrix. *(4 marks)*
Break down the question: there are two clear aspects to this question, the position and the function of the Matrix. Ensure you answer both parts. You have also been asked to 'describe'. This means the examiner wants factual detail, not a one-word answer.

Answer: 'The matrix is found at the proximal end of the nail. It extends from under the nail root to the distal part of the lunula. The function of the matrix is the formation of new nail cells by its germinal zone.'
This question is worth four marks. Always ask yourself, 'Have I provided a clear relevant answer that will attract the maximum marks available?' Look at a badly written answer to the same question and ask yourself how many marks would you award if you were the examiner!

Answer: 'The matrix is found at the base of the nail and it is where the nail cells grow'.
*Yes, it is true the matrix is found at the base of the nail, but so is the lunula and the cuticle – we need to be much more specific. It is also true that this is where the nail cells grow, but the **function** of the matrix is the **formation** or **production** of new nail cells. These are key words that were omitted from this answer.*

Read through these other examples of questions and answers focused around the structure of the nail.

Q1: What is the purpose of the hyponychium, and where is it located?

(2 marks)

Answer: The hyponychium is located under the free edge of the nail where the nail bed and the free edge meet.

The purpose of the hyponychium is protection of the nail bed.

Q2: What is the function of the nail walls, and where are they found?

(2 marks)

Answer: The nail walls are located at the sides of the nail plate. The nail walls frame shape and support the nail plate.

Q3: Where is the cuticle located, what is its function, and how should a healthy cuticle appear? *(3 marks)*

Answer: The cuticle is located around the base of the nail. Its function is to protect the germinal matrix by providing a seal against the outside environment. A healthy cuticle should be soft, free and pliable, without any splits or cracks.

Q4: How does the nail plate adhere to the nail bed? *(4 marks)*

Answer: The surface of the nail bed has an extensive series of longitudinal corrugations that dovetail together with the nail plate to form a strong anchor. The corrugations are more deeply defined closer to the nail walls.

Q5: What is the function and location of the free edge? *(3 marks)*

Answer: The free edge is that part of the nail plate that extends past the hyponychium over the fingertip. The free edge has a protective role, and is the hardest part of the nail. Its location also helps to prevent foreign bodies from entering the nail bed.

Q6: Where are the nail grooves located, and what is their function? *(2 marks)*

Answer: The nail grooves are the deep ridges found between the nail wall and the nail plate. Nail grooves act as tracks along which the growing nail travels as it grows upwards to form the new nail.

Q7: Give two functions of the nail. *(2 marks)*

Answer:
- To protect the end of the finger.
- To assist in precise manipulations, eg lifting of small objects.
- To provide a rigid support for the fingertips.
- To provide a protected area with numerous nerve endings which can enhance a sense of touch.

Some extra points have been provided for you to assist your revision – remember, if a question asks you to provide two points, no extra marks will be awarded if you provide five points.

Q8: Briefly describe the nail plate. *(4 marks)*

Answer: The nail plate is attached firmly to the nail bed by a series of ridges. The nail plate is composed of three scaly layers of dead nerveless cells held together by a minimum amount of moisture (7–12%) and fat. A healthy nail plate should have a semi-transparent, slightly pink appearance. The main role of the nail plate is protection of the delicate areas at the distal part of the fingers and toes.

Q9: What part of the nail is sometimes referred to as the nail body? *(1 mark)*

Answer: This refers to the visible part of the nail plate which is attached to the nail bed.

Q10: What is the lunula, and why is it paler in colour? *(3 marks)*

Answer: The lunula is the pale half moon area at the base of the nail. It is the only visible part of the extended germinal matrix.

The lunula is paler because this part of the germinal matrix is quite thick, so it prevents the healthy glow from the enriched blood supply underneath showing through. The nail plate is less firmly attached in the area of the lunula and this reflects light differently to the rest of the nail body.

Q11: Briefly describe how the nail plate grows and becomes the fully formed nail unit. *(8 Marks)*

Answer: The nail begins its life in the germinal matrix. This area is the reproducing area of the nail. The cells here reproduce by mitosis or cell division. The matrix benefits from an enriched blood supply to assist in this process. As the nail cells move forwards, they undergo keratinisation and become incorporated into the nail plate. This process repeats and repeats, enabling the keratinised cells to move forward over the lunula and along the nail bed to form the nail unit. The nail grooves at the sides of the nail act as 'railway lines' or furrows as the new nail travels forwards. The surface cells of the nail bed also attach to the underside of the growing nail, providing a smooth surface to advance the growing nail.

Q12: Define the phrase 'keratinisation of the nail'. *(1 mark)*

Answer: This is when the nail cells undergo a change to become flat, horny, dead cells without a nucleus.

There is a short self-test at the end of this chapter which includes questions on nail structure.

CONDITIONS OF THE NAIL, HANDS AND FEET

There is often confusion about what is a disease and what is a disorder. Consider the following statements:-

• **Diseases** of the nails, hands and feet cannot be treated by the therapist. They may be contagious and require tactful referral to the clients GP; e.g. paronychia – infection of the tissue around the nail, and tinea pedis – athlete's foot.
• **Disorders** of the nails, hands and feet can be treated by the therapist. They can usually be improved by regular treatment. They are not contagious; eg dry hands and nails and pterygium – forward growth of cuticle.

During training, it is unlikely that you will have the opportunity to come across the many nail diseases and disorders you are required to know about. This is why this area is tested by examination questions.

Examination questions focus on the *appearance* of the condition, its *identifying* factors and the *possible causes*. Look at as many illustrations and photographs as you can to help you to identify various diseases and disorders.

Look at your study notes and the revision maps on pages 46 and 47, then review the model questions and answers. The Revision Maps clearly separate the treatable and non-treatable conditions, and include the commonly seen diseases and disorders.

Revision Map – Some Common Conditions That Should Not Receive Treatment

Severe Onycholysis
- Lifting of nail from its bed at the top or distal end.
- Could be caused by circulation problems or too many nail hardeners.
- Could also be caused by the pressure of ill-fitting shoes.

Paronychia
- Inflammation of the tissues around the nail plate.
- Contagious.
- Painful.
- A bacterial infection.
- Common in people whose hands are frequently in water.

Severe Koilonychia (Spoon nails)
- Appear concave or flat.
- Could be caused by anaemia.
- Could be caused by exposure to harsh chemicals.
- In children it grows out without treatment.
- Could be a congenital condition.

Onychomycosis
- Often called 'ringworm'.
- Affects nail plate and nail bed.
- Yellow, orangey, opaque.
- Crumbly appearance is most common.
- More than one nail is affected.
- Nail lifts from nail bed.
- A fungal infection.

Tinea Pedis
(Athlete's Foot)
- Affects skin of the feet.
- A fungal infection.

Onychia
- Inflammation of the nail bed and matrix.
- A bacterial infection.
- Can follow paronychia.
- Often nail is lost.
- Sometimes trauma initiates this condition.

Impetigo
- Affects skin, not nails.
- Bacterial, contagious.
- Blisters, then crusty.

Eczema
- Itchy.
- Pustular.
- Dry.
- Scaly.
- Red.
- Non-contagious

Psoriasis
- Common.
- Has an unknown cause.
- Large, raised silver plaques.
- Can cause brittle nails and onycholysis.
- Not contagious.

Warts
- A viral infection.
- Affects the hands.
- Infectious to susceptible persons.

Verrucae
- A viral infection.
- Affects plantar surface of feet.
- Infectious to susceptible persons.

Revision Map – Some Conditions or Disorders that can be Improved by Treatment

Onychorrhexis
- Dry split brittle nails.
- Often longitudinal ridges indicates illness.

- Hot oil.
- Thermal mitts.
- Paraffin wax.

Ridged nails
- Normally linked with uneven growth at the matrix.

- Regular manicure.
- Hot oil manicure.
- Extra careful cuticle work.

Pterygium
- Forward and excessive growth of the cuticle.

- Hot oil treatments.
- Regular manicures.
- Regular use of rich moisturisers in a home care routine.

Dry brittle nails
- Caused by:
  - Poor circulation.
  - Chemical agents.
  - Not wearing gloves.

- Hot oil treatments.
- Paraffin wax treatments.
- Thermal mitts and bootees good for improving circulation.
- Massage.
- Regular use of rich moisturisers.

Hangnails
- A break or tear in the tissues of the nail wall.
- Proceed with care.
- Advise client to keep hands well moisturised.

Onychophagy
- Nail biting.

- Have regular manicures.
- Client will probably need a nail strengthener.

Leuconychia
- White spots which grow out.
- Could be caused by poor manicure techniques or trauma.
- More common in women and on the hands.

Beau's Lines
- A transverse line across the nail.
- Caused by trauma or shock.
- Caused also by a temporary retardation of growth which gives the line effect.
- Beau's lines grow out.

Dry hands and feet (anhidrosis)
- Poor circulation is a common cause.
- Overuse of chemical agents, eg detergents.
- Adverse weather conditions can contribute to this condition.

MULTIPLE CHOICE QUESTIONS

The questions below cover *appearance*, *location* and *causes* of a range of conditions. These are vital revision points for you.

When you are revising, try and learn about a good range of diseases and disorders. Carefully consider the descriptions provided before choosing your answer. Only one answer is correct. Indicate your answer by putting an **X** in the circle: ◯

EXAMPLE QUESTION
The nail condition leukonychia is described as:

a) an infectious condition affecting the nail plate ◯

b) an infectious condition affecting the nail bed ◯

c) a non-infectious condition affecting the nail plate ⊗

d) a non-infectious condition affecting the nail wall ◯

Correct answer is **c)**

On completion of the test, check your answers on page 51. It may also help you to visit your college library where examples of previous multi-choice papers may be held. By looking at as many questions as you can, you will gain confidence in preparation for any multi-choice tests you have to take.

Q1. **The condition known as 'blue nails':**

a) affects children only and is a condition where the nails have a bluish tinge caused by a heart condition ◯

b) affects both sexes and is a condition where the nails have a bluish tinge caused by a lack of oxygen, often associated with poor circulation ◯

c) affects both sexes, is caused by circulatory disorders, and is a condition where some of the nails are affected ◯

d) affects children only and is a condition where the nails have a bluish tinge caused by lack of oxygen ◯

Q2. Paronychia is a nail condition which:

a) affects the nail wall, is contagious and caused by bacteria ○

b) affects the nail bed and matrix, is contagious and caused by
bacteria ○

c) affects the nail wall, is non-contagious and is caused by a virus ○

d) affects the nail bed and matrix, is non-contagious and caused by
a virus ○

Q3. Pterygium is a nail disorder which:

a) appears as cracked, split cuticles. The condition improves with
regular manicure. ○

b) appears as excessive overgrowth of the cuticle adhered to the
nail plate. The condition improves with regular manicure ○

c) appears as a ragged and bitten-back free edge. The condition
improves with regular manicure ○

d) appears as tiny pits all over the surface of the nail. The condition
improves with regular manicure ○

Q4. Onycholysis is a nail disorder:

a) identifiable by a lifting of the nail plate caused by incorrect
shaping of the nail ○

b) identifiable by a lifting of the nail plate which always has a
thickened appearance and is more common on the feet ○

c) identifiable by a lifting of the nail plate from the nail bed, is seen
as a pale, even, white area, and is more common on the feet ○

d) identifiable by a lifting of the nail plate from the nail bed, is seen
as a pale, even, white area, and is more common on the hands. ○

Q5. The condition known as onychomycosis is:

a) a bacterial infection which appears as discoloration, lifting,
even crumbling of the nail plate ○

b) a fungal infection which appears as longitudinal ridges on the
nail plate ○

c) a bacterial infection which appears as longitudinal ridges and
increased curvature of the nail plate ○

d) a fungal infection which appears as discoloration, lifting, even
crumbling of the nail plate ○

Q6. The nail condition known as koilonychia is alternatively called:

a) bitten nails ◯

b) corrugated nails ◯

c) ingrown nails ◯

d) spoon nails ◯

Q7. Onychogryptosis is a nail condition:

a) which is infectious, is more common on the feet, and is identifiable by a thickened nail appearance ◯

b) which is non-infectious, often caused by ill-fitting shoes and is commonly called an ingrowing nail ◯

c) which appears as thin, fragile nails which split easily and have a non-lustrous appearance ◯

d) which appears as a series of horizontal ridges across the nail plate, and is non-contagious ◯

Q8. The condition known as leukonychia is:

a) attributed to trauma and possibly poor use of manicure tools; it appears as white spots or lines within the nail plate ◯

b) attributed to iron deficiency or chronic illness; it appears as brown pigmentation under the nail plate ◯

c) attributed to fungal infection; it appears as white spots, and a manicure/pedicure should be avoided ◯

d) attributed to minor trauma, it appears as tiny pits all over the nail with a white undertone. ◯

Q9. The condition known as verruca plantaris:

a) is non-contagious and affects the fingers ◯

b) is contagious between certain individuals and affects the plantar surface of the foot or feet ◯

c) is contagious between certain individuals and affects the palmar surface of the hand or hands ◯

d) is non-contagious and affects the plantar surface of the foot or feet ◯

Q10. The skin condition psoriasis:

a) appears as raised, rough, red areas with a covering of silvery scales. It is non-infectious and affects the sufferer's nails in many cases ○

b) appears as a formation of circles, which dry up leaving yellow scabs. It does not affect the nails ○

c) appears as smooth red patches with a covering of silver scales. The sufferer's nails are never affected ○

d) appears as red pimples which form red circles with a normal skin colour in the centre. It is contagious and can affect the nails in many cases ○

MULTIPLE CHOICE TEST – ANSWERS

1.	B
2.	A
3.	B
4.	C
5.	D
6.	D
7.	B
8.	A
9.	B
10.	A

Marking and Grading

10 correct excellent, superb

8 correct very good

6 correct OK, but go back to your notes and revision guide

Under 5 You need to go back and spend some time revising

PRODUCTS, TOOLS AND EQUIPMENT

As a professional, you are expected to have an understanding of the typical cosmetic ingredients of manicure and pedicure products, and to be able to use tools and equipment effectively. It will help you to learn a basic list of solvents and a basic list of moisturising ingredients. Remember perfume and water are common ingredients included in the manufacture of many products.

Some common solvents
- Amyl acetate
- Butyl acetate
- Ethyl acetate

Some common moisturising ingredients
- Glycerine or glycerol
- Lanolin
- Mineral oil
- Vegetable oil
- Coconut oil
- Cocoa butter
- Beeswax

Review the following Revision Maps, short answer questions, and then attempt the short test at the end of this section.

SHORT ANSWER QUESTIONS

An example of some model questions and answers are provided, to help give you an insight on how to answer questions properly. Reading through the questions and answers will also help your revision. Remember to break down the question into its separate parts.

Q1: **What type of product is cuticle remover, and what is its active ingredient?**

(2 marks)

Answer: Cuticle remover is an alkaline or caustic product. Its active ingredient is 2–5% potassium hydroxide.

Revision Map –
Common Ingredients in Manicure and Pedicure Products

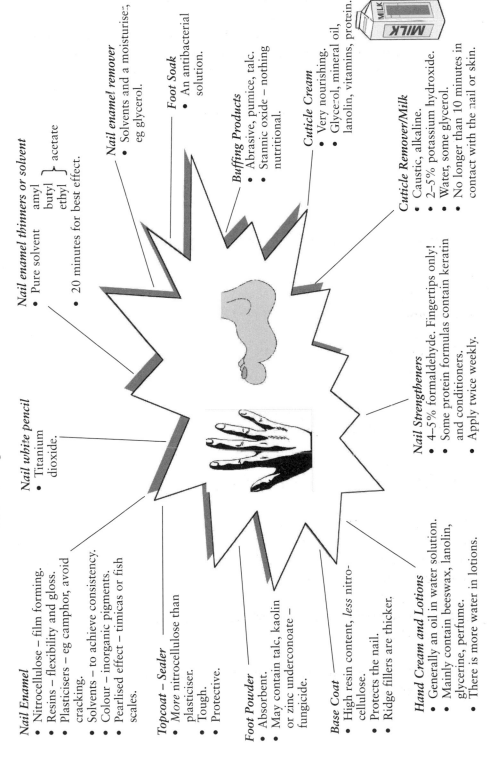

Nail enamel thinners or solvent
- Pure solvent — amyl, butyl, ethyl } acetate
- 20 minutes for best effect.

Nail enamel remover
- Solvents and a moisturiser, eg glycerol.

Foot Soak
- An antibacterial solution.

Buffing Products
- Abrasive, pumice, talc.
- Stannic oxide – nothing nutritional.

Cuticle Cream
- Very nourishing.
- Glycerol, mineral oil, lanolin, vitamins, protein.

Cuticle Remover/Milk
- Caustic, alkaline.
- 2–5% potassium hydroxide.
- Water, some glycerol.
- No longer than 10 minutes in contact with the nail or skin.

Nail Strengtheners
- 4–5% formaldehyde. Fingertips only!
- Some protein formulas contain keratin and conditioners.
- Apply twice weekly.

Hand Cream and Lotions
- Generally an oil in water solution.
- Mainly contain beeswax, lanolin, glycerine, perfume.
- There is more water in lotions.

Base Coat
- High resin content, *less* nitro-cellulose.
- Protects the nail.
- Ridge fillers are thicker.

Foot Powder
- Absorbent.
- May contain talc, kaolin or zinc underconoate – fungicide.

Topcoat – Sealer
- *More* nitrocellulose than plasticiser.
- Tough.
- Protective.

Nail Enamel
- Nitrocellulose – film forming.
- Resins – flexibility and gloss.
- Plasticisers – eg camphor, avoid cracking.
- Solvents – to achieve consistency.
- Colour – inorganic pigments.
- Pearlised effect – timicas or fish scales.

Nail white pencil
- Titanium dioxide.

Revision Map – Tools and Equipment for Nail Treatments of the Hands

Tools and Equipment for Nail Treatments of the hands

Cuticle knife
- Removes any cuticle stuck to the nail plate.
- Sterilise in glass bead or autoclave.
- Keep blade sharp.
- *Never use to cut.*

Cuticle nippers
- Used to clip hangnails.
- Oil mechanism occasionally.
- Sterilise in glass bead or autoclave.

Orangewood Sticks
- Hoofed end for easing back cuticles (always cover).
- Pointed end for cleaning up enamel and removing products from jars.
- Absorbent, so difficult to sterilise.
- Give to client or scrub, rinse and place in UV cabinet.

Nail brush
- Used to remove traces of products from the nails.
- Sterilise by washing, and submerge in chlorahexadine-type solution.

Emery board
- Flexible, long.
- Rough side to reduce length.
- Fine side to smooth free edge.
- Difficult to sterilise properly.
- If re-used, place in UV steriliser between appointments, 15 minutes each side.

Nail scissors
- Used to reduce nail length.
- Sterilise in autoclave or glass bead steriliser

Thermal mitts
- Electrically heated mitts.
- Warmth aids in penetration of products and arthritic pain.
- Follow manufacturer's instructions for use.

Paraffin wax heater
- For providing paraffin wax baths.
- Working temperature maintained at 53°.
- Always include heater in health and safety checks.

Nail buffer
- Increases blood flow.
- Used to buff and shine the nail.
- Chamois leather cover can be removed for washing or replacement.
- Only buff towards the free edge.

Revision Map – Tools and Equipment for Nail Treatments of the Feet

Tools and Equipment for Nail Treatments of the Feet (central)

Cuticle knife
- Remove any cuticle stuck to the nail plate.
- Often a lot of excess cuticle on the toe nails.
- Sterilise in autoclave or glass bead.

Cuticle nippers
- Seldom needed on the feet.

Diamond deb file
- Special metal file for shaping toenails.
- Sterilise in autoclave.

Emery board
- For smoothing free edge of the nail.
- Dispose of afterwards.

Orangewood sticks
- Hoofed end for easing back cuticle (always cover).
- Pointed end for cleaning up enamel and removing products from jars.
- Dispose of after use.

Nail clippers
- Strong metal clippers needed to shorten toe nails, which are stronger than fingernails.
- Oil mechanism regularly.
- Sterilise in autoclave.

Foot bath or foot spa
- Thermostatically controlled heater for soaking the feet.
- May have an agitated action to improve circulation.

Foot file
- Abrasive file use to reduce hard skin on the feet.
- Never use on diabetic clients.

Think! Why is the client getting hard skin? If it's excessive advise a visit to a podiatrist.

Nail brush
- Used to remove traces of products from the nails.
- Sterilise by washing, submerge in chlorahexadine-type solution.

Thermal bootees
- Electrically heated bootees.
- Warmth aids in penetration of products and arthritic pain.
- Follow manufacturer's instructions for use.

Paraffin wax heater
- For providing paraffin wax baths.
- Working temperature maintained at 53°.
- Always include heater in health and safety checks.

Rubber gloves
- Optional.
- Does give some protection from resident bacteria on the client's skin.

Toe separators
- Shaped latex.
- Designed to keep the toes still during enamelling (not allowed by all examining bodies).

Q2: In what product is stannic oxide a common ingredient? *(1 mark)*

Answer: Buffing cream or buffing paste.

Q3: Name a common ingredient of nail white pencil. *(1 mark)*

Answer: Titanium dioxide.

Q4: Name two manicure products which may contain gum tragacanth.

(2 marks)

Answer:
- Hand cream.
- Hand lotion.

Q5: Name *one* ingredient found in foot powder, and give reasons why it is used on clients with hyperhydrosis of the feet? *(3 marks)*

Answer: Foot powder is used on clients with hyperhydrosis (excessive perspiration) because it is absorbent, fungicidal, will help to relieve excessive wetness and may even help diminish resulting odour. A typical ingredient is kaolin.

Q6: Why is nail drying spray used at the end of the nail enamel application, and not after the application of each coat of enamel? *(2 marks)*

Answer: Nail drying spray imparts an oily coating to the enamel surface. It protects the nail enamel from knocks and scuffs by its slippery surface. If it was applied after each coat of enamel, the nail enamel would not adhere to the nail plate properly.

Q7: How should nail scissors be sterilised? *(1 mark)*

Answer: In the autoclave or glass bead steriliser.

Q8: What function do cuticle nippers have in the manicure routine? *(2 marks)*

Answer: Cuticle nippers are used to clip hangnails. They can be used in extreme circumstances to remove excess cuticle tissue.

Q9. What effect does buffing with a chamois buffer have on the nail? *(2 marks)*

Answer: Buffing increases blood circulation to the nails. The chamois buffer can be used with a product such as buffing cream to create a shine on the nail plate.

Q10. What is considered a safe working temperature of paraffin wax for application to the hands or feet? *(1 mark)*

Answer: 53°.

Q11. Why are the nails filed from side to centre? *(1 mark)*

Answer: This prevents splitting of the nail layers and flaking at the nail tip.

Q12. When might a thermal manicure treatment be recommended for a client? *(2 marks)*

Answer:
- If the client has dry hands, nails or cuticles.
- If the client suffers from poor circulation.
- To vary the client's treatment routine or to offer a 'deluxe' service.

Q13. Why is the abrasive foot file frequently needed in a pedicure routine? *(2 marks)*

Answer: Many clients present themselves for pedicure with some degree of hard skin on the feet. The foot file has a gentle abrasive action which helps to reduce the hard skin areas.

Q14. Why could rubber gloves be recommended as protective clothing for a pedicurist? *(3 marks)*

Answer: The feet are washed less frequently than the hands, and are covered with socks and shoes most of the time. These factors assist in the multiplication of bacteria on the feet. By wearing rubber gloves, the pedicurist will reduce the risk of cross-infection between clients, and reduce the risk to themselves of contracting something undesirable from the client.

Q15. Give four guidelines that the therapist can follow to maintain good hygiene levels when pedicuring. *(4 marks)*

Answer:
- Ensure equipment has been adequately sterilised before commencing treatment.
- Do not reuse items that are difficult to sterilise fully, eg emery boards.
- Use disposable paper tissue throughout the treatment for drying and wrapping the feet, and to protect normal linen.
- Always use separate towels from the ones used for other salon treatment.

Additional guidelines include:
- Wear protective gloves.
- Use a specially formulated anti-bacterial product to soak the feet.

ANATOMY AND PHYSIOLOGY

Bones and Muscles of the Hand, Forearm, Foot and Lower Leg

In the past there was a lot of emphasis on anatomy and physiology in beauty therapy courses.

The anatomy and physiology that therapists now need to know at level 2 is based around *awareness*: the beauty therapist must be *aware* of the underlying anatomical structures of the area they are working on.

The Revision Maps provide some essential anatomy you need to know when providing nail treatments, hand and arm massage, and foot and leg massage.

Review your course notes, Revision Maps and the sample questions and answers provided for you.

Blood circulation to the hands and feet

A simple outline of blood circulation to the hands and feet is presented on the Revision Maps on pages 66–69.

You should know about the effects which massage has on the limbs; these points and the important contra-indications are also contained on the Revision Maps.

Revision Map – Bones of the Hand and Forearm

Think about the movement of the hands:
- Joints enable movement. All these joints are synovial.
- The thumb has a special joint, a saddle joint.

*Remember!   S for Special
             S for Saddle*

Without this joint the thumb would be claw-like.
- The fingers or phalanges are hinge joints.
- The wrist or carpus is made up of bones that glide over each other.

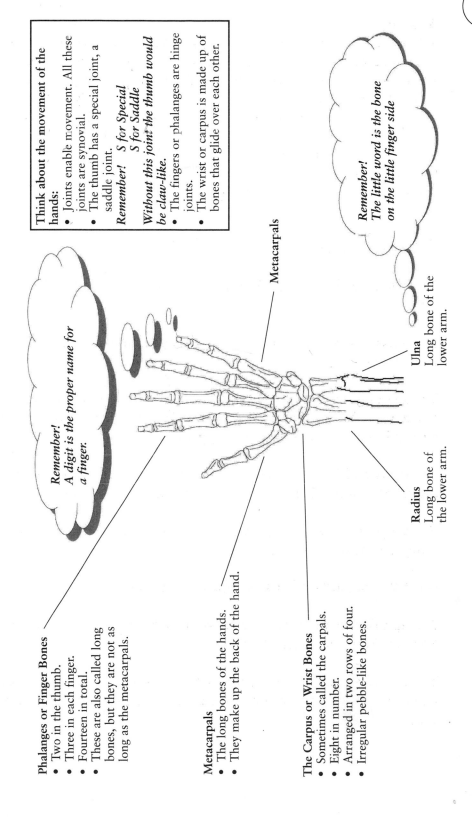

*Remember!
A digit is the proper name for a finger.*

*Remember!
The little word is the bone on the little finger side*

Metacarpals

Ulna
Long bone of the lower arm.

Radius
Long bone of the lower arm.

Phalanges or Finger Bones
- Two in the thumb.
- Three in each finger.
- Fourteen in total.
- These are also called long bones, but they are not as long as the metacarpals.

Metacarpals
- The long bones of the hands.
- They make up the back of the hand.

The Carpus or Wrist Bones
- Sometimes called the carpals.
- Eight in number.
- Arranged in two rows of four.
- Irregular pebble-like bones.

Revision Map – Introductory Muscles of the Hand and Forearm

Palm up

Palm Down

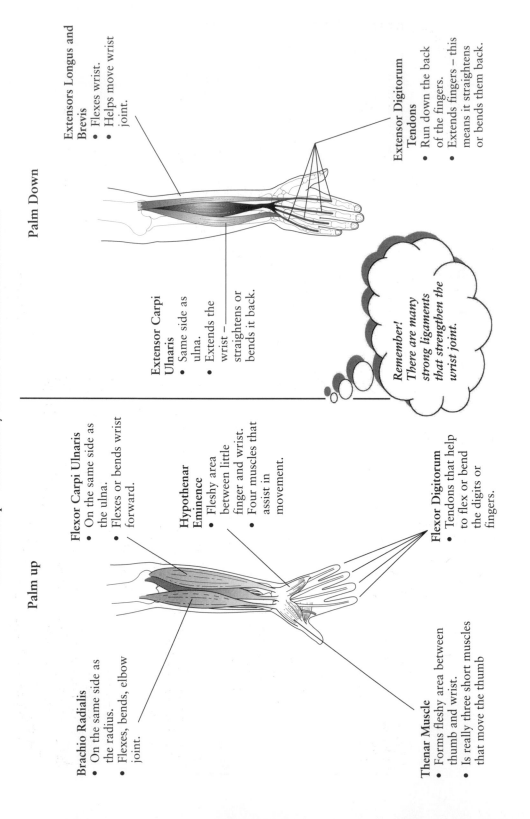

Extensors Longus and Brevis
- Flexes wrist.
- Helps move wrist joint.

Extensor Digitorum Tendons
- Run down the back of the fingers.
- Extends fingers – this means it straightens or bends them back.

Extensor Carpi Ulnaris
- Same side as ulna.
- Extends the wrist – straightens or bends it back.

Remember! There are many strong ligaments that strengthen the wrist joint.

Brachio Radialis
- On the same side as the radius.
- Flexes, bends, elbow joint.

Flexor Carpi Ulnaris
- On the same side as the ulna.
- Flexes or bends wrist forward.

Hypothenar Eminence
- Fleshy area between little finger and wrist.
- Four muscles that assist in movement.

Thenar Muscle
- Forms fleshy area between thumb and wrist.
- Is really three short muscles that move the thumb

Flexor Digitorum
- Tendons that help to flex or bend the digits or fingers.

Revision Map – Bones of the Foot and Lower Leg

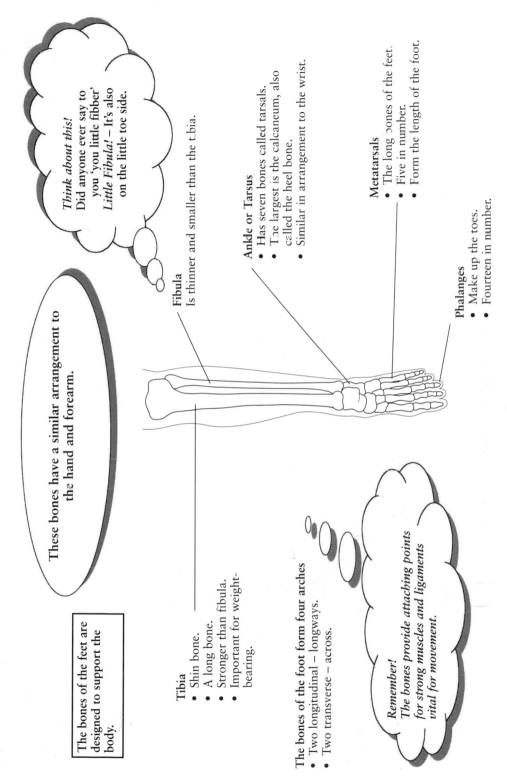

The bones of the feet are designed to support the body.

These bones have a similar arrangement to the hand and forearm.

Think about this!
Did anyone ever say to you 'you little fibber'
Little Fibula! – It's also on the little toe side.

Fibula
Is thinner and smaller than the tibia.

Ankle or Tarsus
- Has seven bones called tarsals.
- The largest is the calcaneum, also called the heel bone.
- Similar in arrangement to the wrist.

Metatarsals
- The long bones of the feet.
- Five in number.
- Form the length of the foot.

Phalanges
- Make up the toes.
- Fourteen in number.

Tibia
- Shin bone.
- A long bone.
- Stronger than fibula.
- Important for weight-bearing.

The bones of the foot form four arches
- Two longitudinal – longways.
- Two transverse – across.

Remember!
The bones provide attaching points for strong muscles and ligaments vital for movement.

Revision Map – Introducing Muscles of the Lower Leg and Foot

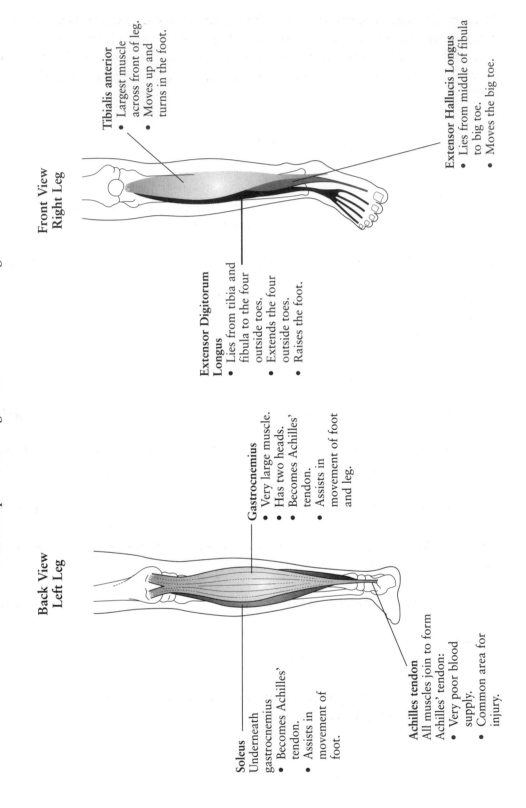

**Front View
Right Leg**

Tibialis anterior
- Largest muscle across front of leg.
- Moves up and turns in the foot.

Extensor Hallucis Longus
- Lies from middle of fibula to big toe.
- Moves the big toe.

Extensor Digitorum Longus
- Lies from tibia and fibula to the four outside toes.
- Extends the four outside toes.
- Raises the foot.

**Back View
Left Leg**

Gastrocnemius
- Very large muscle.
- Has two heads.
- Becomes Achilles' tendon.
- Assists in movement of foot and leg.

Soleus
Underneath gastrocnemius
- Becomes Achilles' tendon.
- Assists in movement of foot.

Achilles tendon
All muscles join to form Achilles' tendon:
- Very poor blood supply.
- Common area for injury.

To help with your understanding of the theory of massage and classification of massage movements you should review Chapter 4. This is about facial massage, and covers everything you need to revise about massage. Some short answer questions around circulation to the limbs follow at the end of this section.

SHORT ANSWER QUESTIONS

An example of some model questions and answers are provided to help give you an insight on how to answer questions properly. Reading through the questions and answers will also help your revision.

Q1. Give a simple description of the ulna bone.   *(4 marks)*

Answer:
- It is found in the lower forearm.
- It is a long bone.
- It is on the same side as the little finger.
- It is longer than the radius.

Q2. Where are the metacarpal bones found?   *(2 marks)*

Answer: They are the long bones of the hand. There are five bones which run from the wrist to the knuckle.

Q3. What is the carpus?   *(2 marks)*

Answer: This is the name given collectively to the wrist bones. There are eight wrist bones or carpals, roughly arranged in two rows of four.

Q4. Give a simple description of the tibia.   *(4 marks)*

Answer:
- The tibia is found in the lower leg.
- It is a long bone.
- It is stronger than the other bone of the lower leg called the fibula.
- It is a weight-bearing bone.

Q5. How many phalanges are there? *(1 mark)*

Answer: There are 14 phalanges in each hand and each foot.

Q6. Give an alternative name for the finger. *(1 mark)*

Answer: A digit.

Q7. Give an alternative name for the pollex. *(1 mark)*

Answer: The thumb.

Q8. Which bone is commonly known as the heel bone? *(1 mark)*

Answer: The calcaneum.

Q9. How many metatarsals are there? Where are these bones? *(3 marks)*

Answer: The metatarsals are the long bones of the feet, and there are five on each foot. They are situated between the ankles and the toes and make up the length of the foot.

Q10. Which bones are known as the tarsals, and where are they found?

(2 marks)

Answer: The tarsals is the name given collectively to the ankle bones. There are seven ankle bones, and they are found at the back of the foot. They form the heel and ankle.

Q11. How many arches are found in the foot? Why are they there? *(3 marks)*

Answer: There are four arches. Two transverse arches and two longitudinal arches. The arches assist in the natural movement of the foot and the support of body weight.

Q12. What are the flexors? *(1 mark)*

Answer: Flexors are muscles that bend forward the body parts they are attached to.

Q13. What are extensors? *(1 mark)*

Answer: Extensors straighten or bend backwards the body parts they are attached to.

Q14. Why do flexors and extensors work together in the lower arm? *(2 marks)*

Answer: The function of the lower arm and hand demand a large range of movement from the muscles in place. Muscles in this area work together to provide this range of movement.

Q15. Describe the thenar eminence. *(2 marks)*

Answer: The thenar eminence is the fleshly part of the hand between the base of the thumb and the wrist. The thenar eminence consists of three short muscles that assist in the movement of the thumb.

Q16. The wrist joint is said to be a strong unit. How is this so? *(3 marks)*

Answer: The wrist joint is made up of eight bones that lie simply in two rows of four. The small bones are able to glide over each other. The wrist joint is strengthened by four main ligaments which give attachment to the strong long bones of the lower arm.

Q17. What is a tendon? *(1 mark)*

Answer: A tendon is an extension of the muscle that attaches a muscle to bone.

Q18. What are ligaments? *(1 mark)*

Answer: Ligaments are the tissues that hold bones to bones.

Q19. What is a synovial joint? *(4 marks)*

Answer: Synovial joints are freely moveable joints which contain a lubricating fluid called Synovial Fluid. The surfaces of the bones in the synovial joint are covered in a slippery cartilage called hyaline cartilage. The joint is held together and secured by a strong protective joint capsule.

66

Revision Map – Blood Supply to the Hand

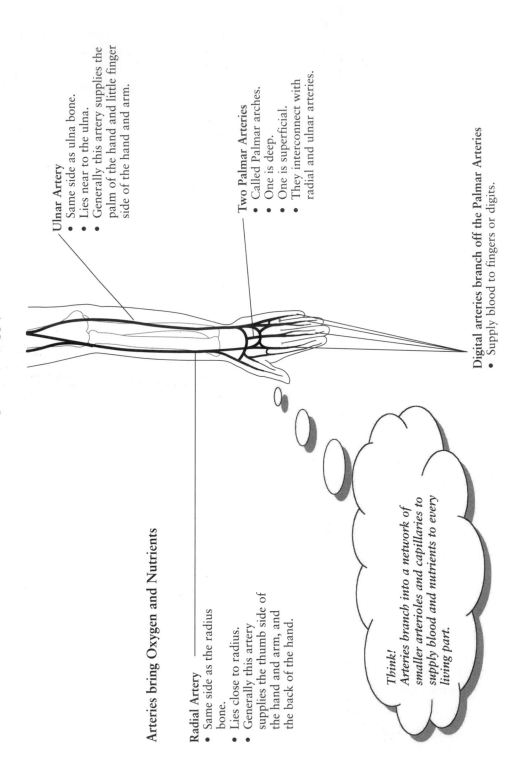

Ulnar Artery
- Same side as ulna bone.
- Lies near to the ulna.
- Generally this artery supplies the palm of the hand and little finger side of the hand and arm.

Two Palmar Arteries
- Called Palmar arches.
- One is deep.
- One is superficial.
- They interconnect with radial and ulnar arteries.

Digital arteries branch off the Palmar Arteries
- Supply blood to fingers or digits.

Arteries bring Oxygen and Nutrients

Radial Artery
- Same side as the radius bone.
- Lies close to radius.
- Generally this artery supplies the thumb side of the hand and arm, and the back of the hand.

Think!
Arteries branch into a network of smaller arterioles and capillaries to supply blood and nutrients to every living part.

Revision Map – Venous Return of the Hand and Arm

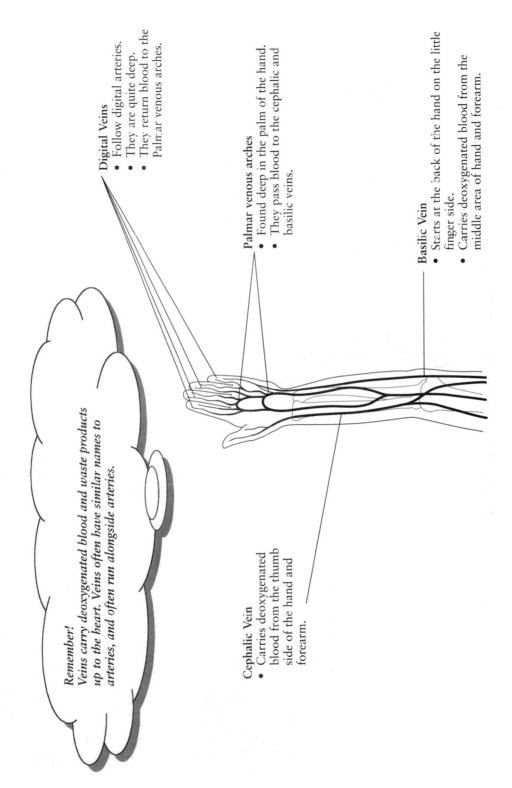

Remember!
Veins carry deoxygenated blood and waste products up to the heart. Veins often have similar names to arteries, and often run alongside arteries.

Digital Veins
- Follow digital arteries.
- They are quite deep.
- They return blood to the Palmar venous arches.

Palmar venous arches
- Found deep in the palm of the hand.
- They pass blood to the cephalic and basilic veins.

Basilic Vein
- Starts at the back of the hand on the little finger side.
- Carries deoxygenated blood from the middle area of hand and forearm.

Cephalic Vein
- Carries deoxygenated blood from the thumb side of the hand and forearm.

Revision Map – Blood Supply to the Foot and Lower Leg

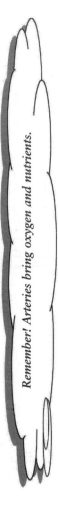

Remember! Arteries bring oxygen and nutrients.

**Front View
Right Leg**

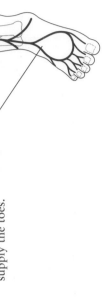

Anterior Tibial Artery
- Lies between the tibia and fibula.
- Passes over the ankle and over the top of the foot.
- The part over the top of the foot is called the dorsalis pedis artery.
- Branches of this artery supply the toes.

**Back View
Right Leg**

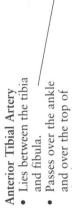

The popliteal artery divides in two just below the knee at the back of the leg.

Posterior Tibial Artery
- Lies down the middle of the leg.
- Passes over the ankle at the back to the sole of the foot.
- Branches supply the heel or calcaneum.
- Under the foot, the artery divides into two to supply the arches of the foot and the toes.

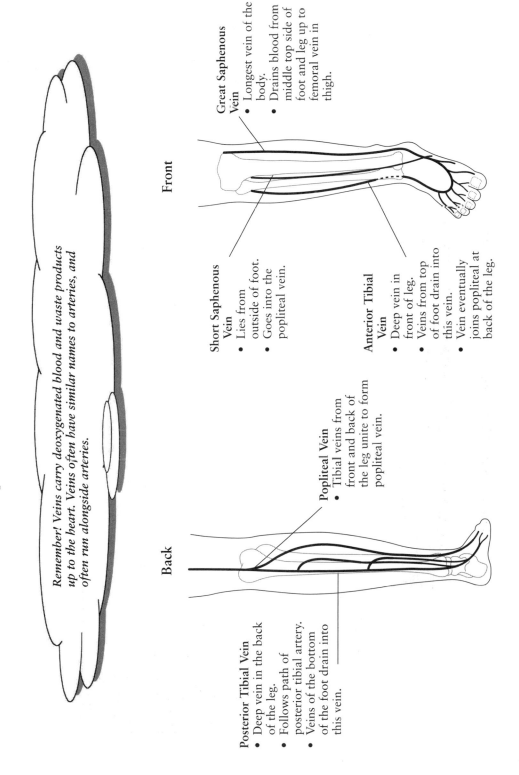

Revision Map – Main Venous Return of the Foot and Lower Limb

Remember! Veins carry deoxygenated blood and waste products up to the heart. Veins often have similar names to arteries, and often run alongside arteries.

Front

Great Saphenous Vein
- Longest vein of the body.
- Drains blood from middle top side of foot and leg up to femoral vein in thigh.

Short Saphenous Vein
- Lies from outside of foot.
- Goes into the popliteal vein.

Anterior Tibial Vein
- Deep vein in front of leg.
- Veins from top of foot drain into this vein.
- Vein eventually joins popliteal at back of the leg.

Back

Popliteal Vein
- Tibial veins from front and back of the leg unite to form popliteal vein.

Posterior Tibial Vein
- Deep vein in the back of the leg.
- Follows path of posterior tibial artery.
- Veins of the bottom of the foot drain into this vein.

Revision Map – Effects of Hand, Arm, Foot and Leg Massage

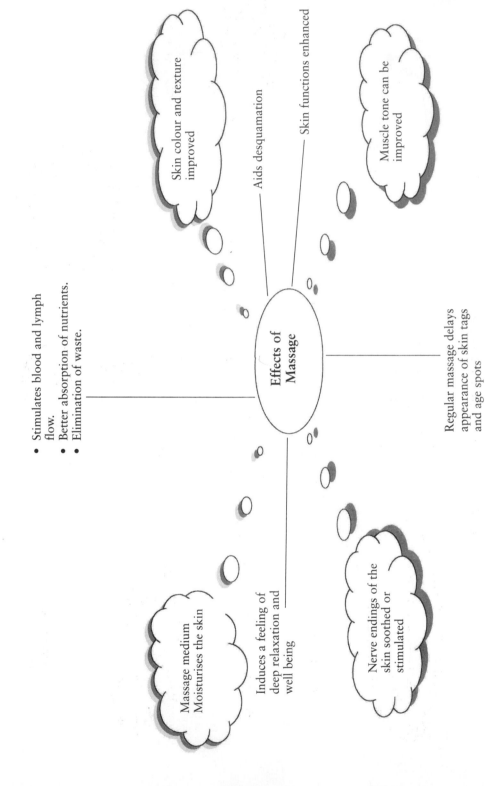

- Stimulates blood and lymph flow.
- Better absorption of nutrients.
- Elimination of waste.

Skin colour and texture improved

Aids desquamation

Skin functions enhanced

Muscle tone can be improved

Effects of Massage

Regular massage delays appearance of skin tags and age spots

Massage medium Moisturises the skin

Induces a feeling of deep relaxation and well being

Nerve endings of the skin soothed or stimulated

Revision Map – General Contra-indications to Massage of the Limbs

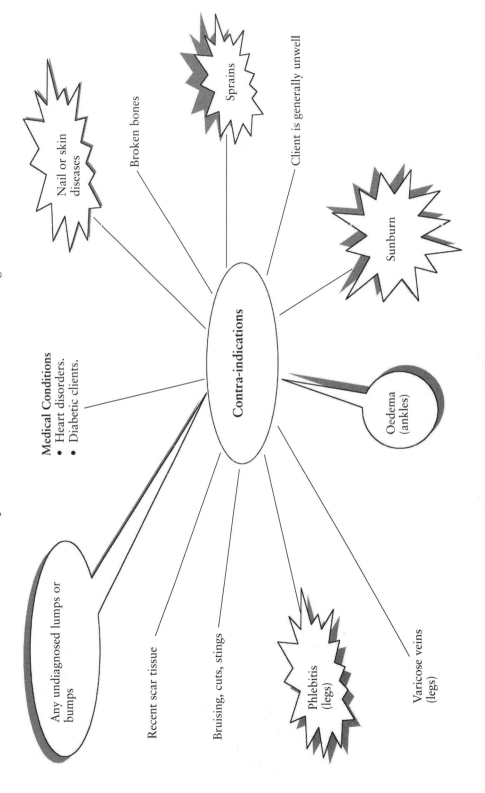

Nail or skin diseases

Broken bones

Sprains

Client is generally unwell

Sunburn

Medical Conditions
- Heart disorders.
- Diabetic clients.

Contra-indications

Oedema (ankles)

Any undiagnosed lumps or bumps

Recent scar tissue

Bruising, cuts, stings

Phlebitis (legs)

Varicose veins (legs)

SHORT ANSWER QUESTIONS

An example of some model questions and answers are provided to help give you an insight on how to answer questions properly. Reading through the questions and answers will also help your revision.

Q1. Briefly explain the arterial blood supply from the lower arm to the nail.

(5 marks)

Answer: There are two main arteries of the lower arm: the ulnar artery and the radial artery. They lie quite close to the ulna and radius bones, from which they take their names. These arteries pass over the wrist area where they form two arches situated in the palm of the hand. The arches are called the palmar arches; one is more superficial than the other.

The palmar arches have branches which supply the fingers; these branches are called the digital arteries. Small branches from the digital arteries supply the nail.

Q2. Which artery is found directly at the back of the knee? *(1 mark)*

Answer: The popliteal artery.

Q3. Where is the dorsalis pedis artery found? *(1 mark)*

Answer: Along the top of the foot.

Q4. Where is the anterior tibial artery found? *(2 marks)*

Answer: The anterior tibial artery is found on the front of the lower leg between the tibia and fibula. It passes over the ankle and then the top of the foot.

Q5. Where is the cephalic vein situated? What is its function? *(2 marks)*

Answer: The cephalic vein is situated in the lower forearm. It carries deoxygenated blood and waste brought from the digital veins, palmar arches and the thumb side of the hand and forearm on its journey back to the heart.

Q6. What are the effects of massage on the lower legs and feet? *(4 marks)*

Answer: Massage increases blood and lymph flow which will aid elimination and absorption in the area being treated.

Massage aids desquamation and improves the colour and texture of the skin. On the lower limbs and feet which carry the weight of the body it can be an especially soothing, beneficial treatment. The massage medium will also moisturise the skin.

Q7. Name three contra-indications that would prevent a hand and arm treatment from being carried out. *(3 marks)*

Answer:
- If a nail disease was present.
- If a skin disease was present.
- A recent fracture or sprain.

Q8. Name six contra-indications to a foot and leg massage treatment. *(6 marks)*

Answer:
- If a nail disease was present.
- If a skin disease was present.
- A recent fracture or sprain.
- Excessive oedema.
- A varicose vein condition.
- Phlebitis.

MAINTAINING HYGIENE LEVELS AND A SAFE WORKING ENVIRONMENT

The following Revision Maps will emphasis the key points you should uphold during nail treatments.

This topic is more realistically monitored and assessed in the practical situation.

Further information, Revision Maps and model questions and answers regarding hygiene, health and safety can be found in Chapter 1.

Revision Map – Maintaining Hygiene – Nail Treatments

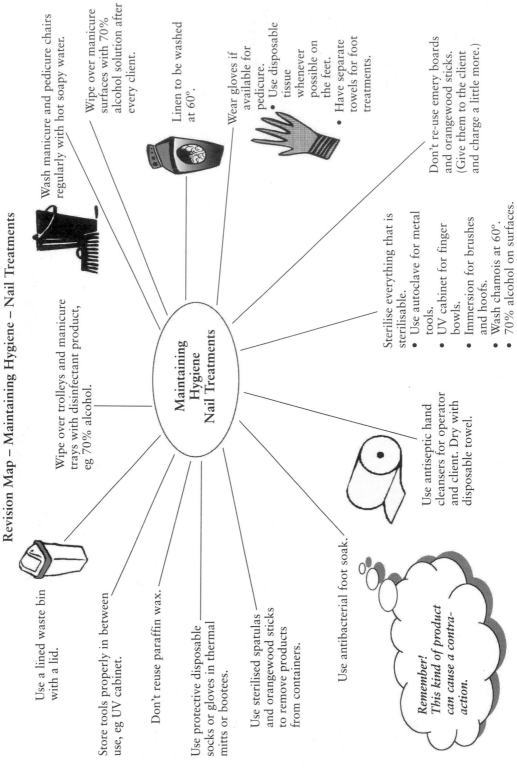

Maintaining
Hygiene
Nail Treatments

Wash manicure and pedicure chairs regularly with hot soapy water.

Wipe over manicure surfaces with 70% alcohol solution after every client.

Linen to be washed at 60°.

Wear gloves if available for pedicure.

- Use disposable tissue whenever possible on the feet.
- Have separate towels for foot treatments.

Don't re-use emery boards and orangewood sticks. (Give them to the client and charge a little more.)

Sterilise everything that is sterilisable.
- Use autoclave for metal tools.
- UV cabinet for finger bowls.
- Immersion for brushes and hoofs.
- Wash chamois at 60°.
- 70% alcohol on surfaces.

Use antiseptic hand cleansers for operator and client. Dry with disposable towel.

Use antibacterial foot soak.

Use sterilised spatulas and orangewood sticks to remove products from containers.

Use protective disposable socks or gloves in thermal mitts or bootees.

Don't reuse paraffin wax.

Store tools properly in between use, eg UV cabinet.

Use a lined waste bin with a lid.

Wipe over trolleys and manicure trays with disinfectant product, eg 70% alcohol.

Remember!
This kind of product can cause a contra-action.

74

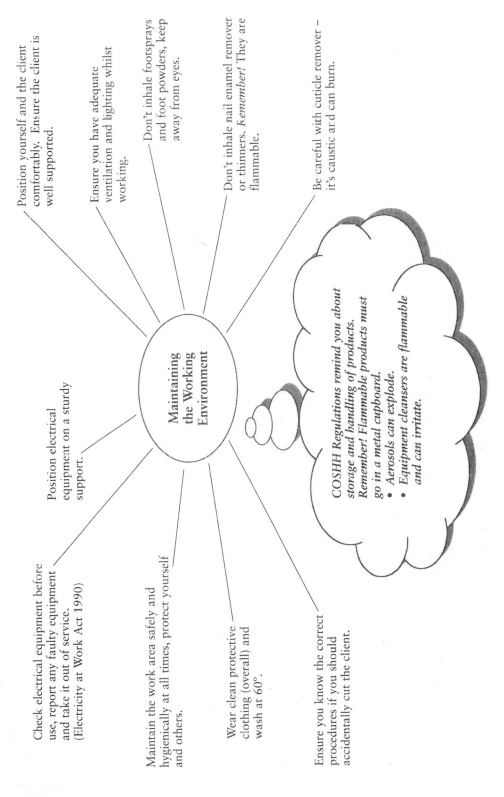

Revision Map – Maintaining the Working Environment

Position yourself and the client comfortably. Ensure the client is well supported.

Ensure you have adequate ventilation and lighting whilst working.

Don't inhale footsprays and foot powders, keep away from eyes.

Don't inhale nail enamel remover or thinners. *Remember!* They are flammable.

Be careful with cuticle remover – it's caustic and can burn.

Position electrical equipment on a sturdy support.

Maintaining the Working Environment

Check electrical equipment before use, report any faulty equipment and take it out of service. (Electricity at Work Act 1990)

Maintain the work area safely and hygienically at all times, protect yourself and others.

Wear clean protective clothing (overall) and wash at 60°.

Ensure you know the correct procedures if you should accidentally cut the client.

COSHH Regulations remind you about storage and handling of products. Remember! Flammable products must go in a metal cupboard.
- *Aerosols can explode.*
- *Equipment cleansers are flammable and can irritate.*

DEVISING TREATMENT PLANS FOR CLIENTS

You should be able to accomplish this task quite naturally and regularly in practical sessions. Sometimes your ability to do this is tested in exams by providing you with 'scenarios' which describe a client and ask you to choose a treatment plan from examples provided. Only *one* treatment plan is correct; the other treatment plans should be eliminated.

Sometimes it will be easy for you to perform the elimination process, because some treatment plans are quite clearly wrong. But at other times it will be difficult, because the treatment plans have been carefully thought out and can be quite tricky. There are basically two things to be done when answering scenario type questions:

1. Look carefully, point by point, at the description of the client. Carefully consider what is required by the client, and ask yourself, 'What are the clients needs?'
2. Systematically look at each stage of the treatment plan and judge for yourself – *yes, this would meet the clients needs and is appropriate,* OR *no, this is not needed and is not appropriate.*

An example of a client scenario and possible treatment plans is provided for you. You will see an attempt has been made to try and fit each step of the treatment plan against the client's requirements. By doing this, it is easier to arrive at the correct answer.

Sample Treatment Plans

Q. Select the most appropriate treatment plan for Mrs Bolland. Only one plan is correct

Ptergyium denotes extra cuticle work.

This means the hands are in water a lot and meet with harsh conditions.

Mrs Bolland
Age 35
occupation Hairdresser
dry cuticles
slight ptergyium
dry hands
soft, short, uneven nails
many hangnails
poor circulation

The dry hands and cuticles will need enriched products. Maybe hot oil or paraffin wax might be appropriate.

These will need careful clipping.

The uneven nails will need careful filing to an appropriate length (as short as the shortest).

This means the hands will have a poor colour, probably bluey. This will influence the choice of enamel. No reds or pinks. Look for other colours. The treatment plan should include something to improve circulation; maybe massage or thermal treatments.

The nails are also soft. This will call for some type of nail strengthener. The shortness of the nails will restrict choice of enamel colour. Nothing too bright or too dark.

By carefully looking point by point at the description of Mrs Bolland's nails, we can actually determine what the client needs.

PLAN A

- Regular routine manicure treatment.

- French style enamel.

This plan offers the client nothing special. The French enamel would not enhance the short nail appearance.
REJECTED!

PLAN B

- Careful filing to even up the nail shape.

Yes – this would meet the client's needs.

- Extra cuticle work using knife nippers and hoof.

Yes – this would meet the client's needs.

- Hand massage with hand lotion.

Hand massage yes – but hand lotion is much too thin for the dry condition.

- Ridge filling basecoat and two coats of enamel in Candy Pink.

This client has soft nails not ridges so ridge-filling basecoat would not be required. The Candy Pink enamel would make the hands look more blue.
REJECTED!

PLAN C

- Hot oil manicure with emphasis on cuticle work.

Yes – this would fit, but there is no mention of any special filing!

- Careful use of knife nippers and hoof.

Yes – this client needs the careful use of manicure tools for the pterygium and hangnails.

- Hand massage with warm oil.

Yes – the warm oil would be a good massage medium for this client.

- Basecoat and two coats of Siren Red enamel.

The red enamel would be inappropriate for the short nails and poor hand colour, also only basecoat is recommended. The client really needs a nail strengthener or hardener.
REJECTED!

PLAN D

- Careful filing to even up the nail shape.

  Yes – this would meet the client's needs.

- Extra cuticle work using knife nippers and hoof.

  Yes – this would meet the client's needs.

- Extended hand massage using a treatment hand cream.

  Yes – this would meet the client's needs and the extended time is positive.

- Application of conditioning and strengthening basecoat.

  Yes – this would meet the client's needs.

- Application of two coats of nail enamel in Nude.

  Yes – this would be appropriate.
  CORRECT!

REMEMBER!

When you are answering scenario type questions, you must select a treatment plan that is the *most appropriate* out of the *options given*, and not necessarily what *you* would have chosen. Many beauty students train in salons or centres that have fantastic manicure and pedicure products, gadgets and machines, while other students receive training in well-equipped but basic salons. Examiners are not allowed to use proprietary names, nor are they allowed to question candidates about specific manicure or pedicure systems.

Some further scenario examples are included for you to review and answer.

The correct answer and a justification follows each scenario.

Q1. Select the most appropriate treatment plan for Mrs Campbell.

A. Plan selected _____

> Mrs Campbell
> Age 40
> Occupation – Florist
> Strong, long, oval nails
> Slight staining of the nails due to constant
> wearing of nail enamel
> Cuticle condition fair
> Hands ingrained, rough and callus on
> thumbs and index finger of right hand
> Skin condition dry
> Enamel must complement an olive green outfit

PLAN A

- Regular shaping and buffing.
- Careful cuticle work with the nail included in the application of cuticle remover.
- Hard skin remover massaged into callused and ingrained area.
- General exfoliation of the hands with exfoliating cream – remove thoroughly.
- Massage with warm oil and apply paraffin wax.
- Wrap carefully.
- On removal of paraffin wax, tissue off residue of oil and perspiration.
- Apply two layers of basecoat.
- Two coats of crème enamel in Soft Peach.

PLAN B

- Regular shaping and buffing.
- Careful cuticle work with the nail included in the application of cuticle remover.
- General exfoliation of the hands with exfoliating cream – remove thoroughly.
- Apply treatment moisturiser, massage and place hands in warm thermal mitts.
- On removal, tissue off any residue.
- Apply two layers of basecoat.
- Apply two layers of clear enamel.

PLAN C

- Regular shaping and buffing.
- Careful cuticle work with the nail included in the application of cuticle remover.
- Hard skin remover massaged into the callused and ingrained area.
- General exfoliation of the hands with an oatmeal scrub.
- Rinse off any residue.
- Extended massage with warm oil.
- Tissue off any residue oil.
- Apply hand cream containing protein.
- Apply all-in-one enamel, two coats in Poppy Red.

Answer: Mrs Campbell: Correct plan = **PLAN A**

PLAN A met all the requirements of Mrs Campbell. Because the nails are stained and the client constantly wears nail enamel, two coats of basecoat were chosen. A Peach enamel would go overall with an olive green outfit, and would not draw attention to the poor condition of the hands.

PLAN B was also a good overall plan for the client, but the clear enamel choice would enable the nail stains to show through. Also, the callused area was not really addressed in the treatment plan.

PLAN C was also a good overall plan with a lot of opportunity to re-moisturise the hands, but the problem lay at the enamel stage. No basecoat was advised and it must be used to prevent further staining, especially with a strong colour like Poppy Red.

Q2. Select the most appropriate treatment plan for Mr Bartlett.

A. Plan Selected _____

> Mr Bartlett
> Age 32
> Occupation – Dentist
> Nails are dry, brittle and short
> Skin of the hands is also dry
> Cuticles are very neglected and overgrown
> Client is prepared to use a home care product
> Time available for treatment is 20 minutes,
> between his morning and afternoon surgery

PLAN A

- Careful filing, retaining a masculine shape.
- Nail soak in hot oil.
- Cuticle work using hoof knife and removal of all excessive overgrown cuticle with nippers.
- Massage with treatment hand cream.
- Application of protein and conditioning nail strengthener.
- Application of clear enamel (two coats).
- Home care product advised is a nail strengthener.

PLAN B

- Careful filing, retaining a masculine shape.
- Nail soak in hot oil.
- Cuticle work using hoof and knife to ease back overgrown cuticles.
- Massage with treatment hand cream.
- Buffing to the nails using buffing paste.
- Home care product advised is an enriched cuticle cream.

PLAN C

- Careful filing, retaining a masculine shape.
- Nail soak in hot oil.
- Cuticle work using hoof knife and nippers if appropriate.
- Massage with warm massage oil.
- Tissue off residue oil.
- Application of basecoat, clear enamel and topcoat.
- Home care product advised is a non-acetone remover to remove enamel.

Answer: Mr Bartlett: Correct plan = **PLAN B**

PLAN B met all the requirements of Mr Bartlett. Medical personnel are not allowed to wear nail enamel during working hours (this also applies to persons working in the catering industry). The buffing aspect of the treatment would have provided a pleasant shine to the nails. The home care product was also a good choice because the nails and cuticles would benefit from enriched cuticle cream.

PLAN A would probably have butchered the client's cuticles. Remember, removing the cuticles could leave the nail fold open to infection. Nail strengthener and clear enamel could also chip and should not be worn by working medical personnel.

PLAN C was also inappropriate in its use of enamel. The home care product would be a poor choice for this client, who clearly needs to have his nails, cuticles and hands re-moisturised.

Q3. Select the most appropriate treatment plan for Mrs Hallmark.

A. Plan Selected _____

> Mrs Hallmark
> Age 60
> Recently retired waitress
> Requires pedicure
> Several callus on plantar surface of the foot
> Several broken veins around ankles
> Thickened toenails
> No signs of any fungal or bacterial infection
> Requires a summer colour enamel

PLAN A

- Regular preparation, washing.
- Cutting of toe nails with spring nippers.
- Filing with crystal coated nail file.
- Regular cuticle work.
- Foot and leg massage using cooling leg balm.
- Great care and light effleurage only around ankles.
- Application of hard skin remover to callused area, massaged in.
- Enamel application in Summer Pink.

PLAN B

- Regular preparation, washing.
- Cutting of toe nails with spring nippers.
- Filing with crystal coated nail file.
- Regular cuticle work.
- Application of hard skin remover to callused area.
- Thorough systematic application of coarse pumice stone to callused area.
- Foot and leg massage using super moisturising product.
- Great care and light effleurage only around ankles.
- Enamel application in Summer Pink.

PLAN C

- Regular preparation, washing.
- Cutting of toe nails with spring nippers.
- Filing with crystal coated nail file.
- Regular cuticle work.
- Using surgical blade, gently remove callus, discard dead skin in sharps box.
- Foot and leg massage with super moisturising product.
- Great care and light effleurage only around ankles.
- Enamel application in Summer Glow.

PLAN D

- Regular preparation, washing.
- Avoid cutting thickened toe nails, file into shape using a coarse emery board.
- Regular cuticle work.
- Using protected surgical blade carefully remove callus, discard dead skin in sharps box.
- Foot and leg massage with cooling leg balm and place feet in thermal bootees for 10 minutes.
- Great care and light effleurage only around ankles.
- Enamel application in Summer Glow.

Answer: Mrs Hallmark: Correct plan = **PLAN B**

PLAN B met all the requirements of Mrs Hallmark, who required quite a regular pedicure. Because of her occupation, the thickened nails could have been caused by pressure perhaps from ill-fitting shoes. No doubt this client walked many miles in a day.

PLAN A was really a bit too basic, and might have been more appropriate as a maintenance type treatment. The big failing with this plan is the fact that no attempt to lessen the callused area was made. The application of hard skin remover will help, but the use of a pumice stone or exfoliating rasp is essential to reduce the thickened skin. Also, bear in mind that callus will need to be reduced over a period of time by the beauty therapist.

PLAN C the main problem here was the use of the surgical blade. Beauty therapists are not advised or generally insured to cut the skin.

PLAN D contains two main errors. The use of the surgical blade and the use of the hot bootees would have been questionable in view of the fact Mrs Hallmark had *several* broken veins around the ankle.

Q4. Select the most appropriate treatment plan for Mrs Bunn.

A. Plan Selected _____

> Mrs Bunn
> Age 50
> Occupation – Teacher
> Requires pedicure
> Complains of aching legs because of standing a lot
> Has a slight arthritic condition
> No callus present but has a corn on the right small toe
> Has a problem with excessively dry skin and nails
> Wants some home care advice

PLAN A

- Regular preparation, washing.
- Soak foot with the addition of strong germicidal product, due to the presence of the corn.
- Regular pedicure procedure, omitting the small right toe.
- Massage with super rich emollient to the foot and ankle only, concentrating on the joints.
- Remove excess product with toner.
- Apply moisturising basecoat.
- Application of enamel of the clients choice.
- Home care advice:
  a) Apply moisturiser regularly.
  b) Use pumice stone during bathing on the corn.
  c) Avoid standing whenever possible.

PLAN B

- Regular preparation, washing.
- Cover corn with plaster.
- Regular pedicure procedure.
- Foot and leg massage with extra rotations to the ankle joint and toes.
- Apply extra layer of moisturiser and place client in thermal bootees.
- Tissue off any excess perspiration.
- Apply base, colour and topcoat.
- Home care advice:
  a) Purchase corn plaster from reputable chemist.
  b) Apply massage oil, eg almond oil, after bathing to the feet and lower legs.
  c) Have regular pedicures and thermal bootee pedicures.

PLAN C

- Regular preparation, washing.
- Foot soak has the addition of a small amount of almond oil.
- Regular pedicure procedure, with careful handling of small right toe.
- Extended massage with moisturising product, leave residue on skin.
- Application of paraffin wax wrap in warm towels.
- Leave until cool.
- Tissue off excess perspiration.
- Apply moisturising basecoat.
- Application of enamel of client choice.
- Advise the client to seek services of podiatrist regarding the corn.
- Home care advice:
  a) Apply heavy moisturiser twice daily.
  b) Attempt to massage moisturiser in, which may help aching legs. Give a short demonstration of a simple massage process.
  c) Have regular paraffin wax treatments.

Answer: Mrs Bunn: Correct plan = **PLAN C**

PLAN C was the only plan that mentioned referral to a podiatrist to address the problem of the corn. The use of paraffin wax is well renowned for the treatment of arthritic conditions and dry skin conditions. This plan also had the addition of a small amount of oil to the foot soak, which would have made the soaking part of the treatment less drying.

PLAN A this plan omitted the toe with the corn, which was quite unnecessary. Excess massage product was removed with toner. This would not be ideal for a client with excessively dry feet, as they would benefit more from the product being left on. There was also no need for the strong germicidal soak – again this was too drying and the presence of a corn is not necessarily a contra-indication. The home care advice in this plan was general. The use of a pumice stone is not totally incorrect, but a beauty therapist should advise the services of another professional and not really the use of a pumice stone.

PLAN B was an average treatment plan, but it would not be necessary to cover the corn with a plaster. It would not be professional to advise the client to visit the local chemist for a remedy corn plaster. The thermal bootees would also have been a suitable treatment for this client.

FINAL END TEST

This section consists of statements. Each one may be correct or incorrect. The answer required is simply

Yes or No.

In your assessment of whether the statement is correct or incorrect, you must only base your answer on the information provided. The questions are arranged in groups in the order that the related topics occurred in the text. After ensuring that all the questions have been answered, check the answers yourself at the back of the chapter.

- FINAL END TEST

1. The cuticle found under the free edge of the nail is the hyponychium.

2. The process of nail growth takes place by cell division in the nail bed.

3. The function of the eponychium or cuticle is protection of the nail fold.

4. The germinal matrix forms the floor of the nail fold.

5. The nail plate adheres to the nail bed by a series of ridges that dovetail together.

6. The nail plate comprises of two layers of keratinised cells.

7. The purpose of the free edge is for protection.

8. The protein found in the nail plate is called keratin.

9. The protective tissue found under the free edge is called the perionychium.

10. The cells of the germinal matrix are similar to the stratum lucidum.

11. Thickened nails *may* be caused by poor arterial supply or a fungal infection.

12. Beau's lines are horizontal ridges across the nail plate and are a definite contra-indication.

13. Nail growth in the toe nail is on average 1 mm per week.

14. Leuconychia rarely results from an illness but is often caused by minor trauma.

15. Koilonychia or spoon nails are more commonly found in the fingernails and are linked with conditions of iron deficiency anaemia.

16. Onychocryptosis or ingrowing nails could be caused by ill-fitting shoes or poor nail cutting techniques.

17. Onychomycosis is not infectious.

18. A fungal infection of the nail plate presents itself as red lines under the nail plate.

19. A fungal infection of the nail plate could be a result of poor personal hygiene.

20. Paronychia is a non-contagious condition that affects the nail wall.

21. Paronychia is characterised by inflammation of the tissues around the nail plate.

22. Extremely dry flaky skin on the feet could be caused by poor arterial circulation.

23. Potassium hydroxide is found in cuticle cream.

24. Hand creams contain less water than hand lotions.

25. Butyl acetate is a common solvent found in nail enamel remover.

26. Cuticle milk is a caustic product.

27. 4–5% formaldehyde is frequently found in nail strengtheners.

28. Beeswax is found in buffing paste.

29. Ridge filling basecoats are thinner than traditional basecoats.

30. Plasticisers are added to nail enamel formulations because they help prevent cracking of the enamel.

31. Topcoat is applied to enhance the life of the enamel applications, and to seal and protect the enamel application.

32. Nail enamel removers should never be used to thin down enamels because they contain a moisturising agent.

33. Arthritic hands would benefit from a paraffin wax treatment.

34. Paraffin wax should be removed from the treatment area when it is still warm.

35. Foot and leg massage should follow the same routine to fit in with the pedicure procedure and time restraints.

36. The beauty therapist should remove callus with a foot rasp or pumice stone and appropriate products.

37. A client with thin fragile nails should be advised during treatment planning to have regular manicures that include the use of a nail strengthener.

38. Thermal pedicures are very useful for clients with aching feet and dry skins.

39. The enamel choice should be decided with the client before the nail treatment begins.

40. If a client presents themselves for a manicure and the cuticles are in a poor condition, the therapist should inform the client that results will take more than one treatment.

41. The humerus is found in the lower arm.

42. The long bones of the hands are the metatarsals.

43. Another name for the pollex is the thumb.

44. The ulna is longer than the radius.

45. The wrist is made up of eight small bones.

46. The tibia is larger than the fibula.

47. There are four arches of the foot.

48. The anatomical name of the heel bone is the calcaneum.

49. The metatarsal phalangial joint is a hinge joint.

50. The digital arteries are found in abundance in the fingers.

51. The brachial artery is found in the lower leg.

52. The posterial tibial artery is the main artery supplying blood to the foot.

53. The deep saphanous vein is found in the upper arm.

FINAL END TEST **ANSWERS**

1. Yes
2. No   This is the matrix.
3. Yes
4. Yes
5. Yes
6. No   It has three layers of dead nerveless keratinized cells.
7. Yes
8. Yes
9. No   The hyponchium.
10. No   They are similar to the germinative layer of the skin.
11. Yes
12. No   Beau's lines do not contra-indicate a manicure but they are horizontal ridges.
13. Yes
14. Yes
15. Yes
16. Yes
17. No   Onychomycosis (or ringworm) is very infectious.
18. No   Often yellow/orangy streaks and crumbly nails are the true appearance.
19. Yes
20. No   Paronychia is very infectious, but it does affect the nail plate.
21. Yes
22. Yes
23. No   It is found in cuticle remover. 2–5%.
24. Yes
25. Yes
26. Yes
27. Yes
28. No   Beeswax is not found in buffing products. They contain abrasive products like talc and stannic oxide.
29. No   They are thicker to fill in the ridges.

30. Yes

31. Yes

32. Yes

33. Yes

34. No   Removal should happen when the wax is cold.

35. No   Foot and leg massage should be applied around the client's needs.

36. Yes   No cutting with surgical blades is to be performed by a beauty therapist.

37. Yes

38. Yes

39. Yes

40. Yes

41. No   The humerus is found in the upper arm. The bones of the lower arm are the radius and ulna.

42. No   The metatarsals are the long bones of the feet. The metacarpals is the correct answer.

43. Yes

44. Yes

45. Yes

46. Yes

47. Yes

48. Yes

49. Yes

50. Yes

51. No   The brachial artery is found in the arm.

52. Yes

53. No   The deep saphanous vein is found in the leg.

Marking Guide and Grading

Check your answers and then look at the guide below. In percentage terms 60% is considered a pass. With this type of end test, because it's a simple Yes or No answer, there is a strong likelihood you could have guessed some of the answers! You should take this into account when determining your grade.

32 correct answers   a pass, well done

42 correct answers   a credit, excellent

Above 48 correct answers is exceptional!

Below 32 correct answers means you need to spend more time revising, so go back to your course notes and Revision Maps, and then have another go.

THE SKIN, SKIN CLEANSING,
EXFOLIATION AND STEAMING

CHECKLIST ✓ Can You?

THE STRUCTURE OF THE SKIN

The beauty therapist must understand the structure and functions of the skin in order to understand how beauty treatments can bring about improvements. The subject of the skin will always be tested thoroughly in assessments or examinations.

Diagrams of the skin

An easy way for the examiner to assess if a student knows about skin structure is to ask the student to draw and label a cross section diagram of the skin, or to label a pre-prepared diagram. Follow this step by step guide: it will take you through the simple stages of building up a clear and accurate diagram.

STEP 1
Review your course notes to give yourself some familiarity of the skins diagramatical appearance.

STEP 2
Remember, you are attempting to draw a technically correct diagram, not produce a masterpiece.

STEP 3
Make the diagram big – use the whole page if you want. Nobody wants to label a tiny diagram, and furthermore the examiner will hate marking it.

STEP 4
Use coloured crayons if it helps you.

STEP 5
Remember, always give the diagram a title.

STEP 6

Draw a hair with a proper shaped base. Give it a label.

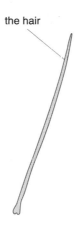

the hair

STEP 7

Provide the hair with a follicle to sit in and a sebaceous gland for lubrication. At this point draw in a skin surface.

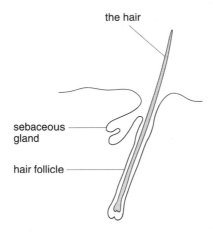

the hair

sebaceous gland

hair follicle

STEP 8
Add a sweat gland that has an opening.

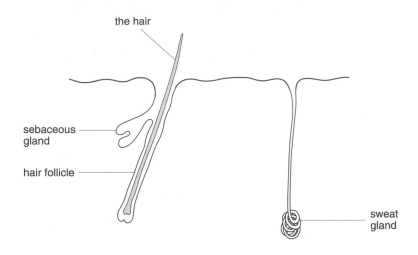

the hair

sebaceous
gland

hair follicle

sweat
gland

STEP 9
Add the dividing line to make the epidermis, and some 'bubbles' to give a subcutis.

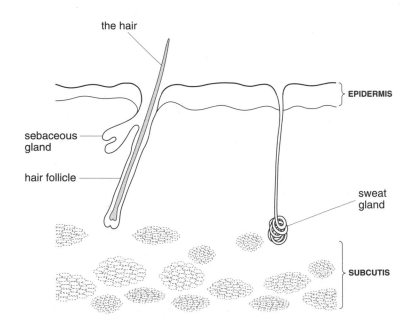

the hair

EPIDERMIS

sebaceous
gland

hair follicle

sweat
gland

SUBCUTIS

STEP 10

Label the dermis and add the arrector pili muscle.

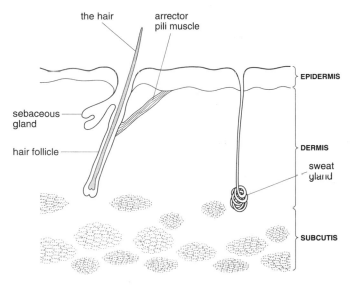

STEP 11

The hardest work is now over! Remember the dermis is the main living area, and contains nerve endings and blood capillaries. To add sensory nerves, think about what your own skin can feel – **heat, cold, pressure, touch.**
Draw in the nerve endings, at different levels.

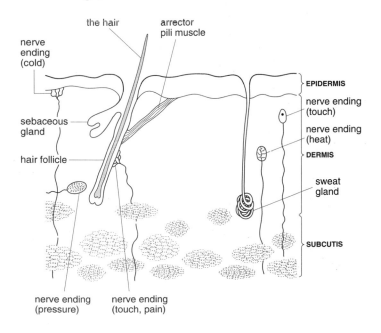

STEP 12

The skin and hair needs a blood supply. For simplicity this could be drawn in red and blue crayons:

- red for arteries and capillaries
- blue for veins and venules

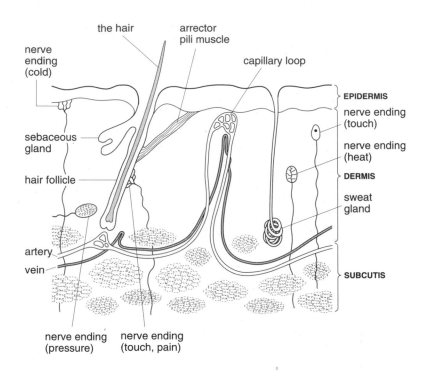

STEP 13

Also found in the dermis are collagen fibres to help maintain the firmness of the skin, and elastin to give elasticity (stretchability). Add these to the diagram, using a simple format.

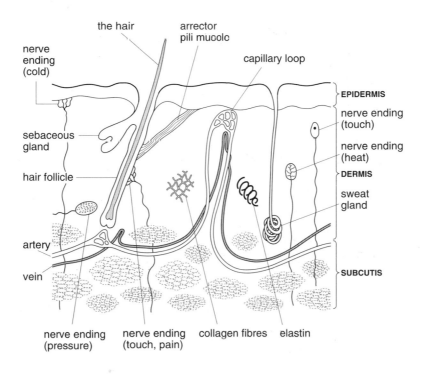

nerve ending (cold)

the hair

arrector pili muscle

capillary loop

EPIDERMIS

nerve ending (touch)

nerve ending (heat)

sebaceous gland

hair follicle

DERMIS

sweat gland

artery

vein

SUBCUTIS

nerve ending (pressure)

nerve ending (touch, pain)

collagen fibres

elastin

The Epidermis

You will need to know about the uppermost layer of the skin: *the epidermis*. The epidermis consists of 5 different cell layers. To add the different cell layers to the skin diagram may overcrowd it, and it would be very difficult to show properly the features of the cell layers in the space allocated. It is logical therefore that examiners will prepare separate questions about the epidermis. A simple way to draw the layers of the epidermis is to use five different coloured crayons.

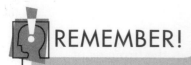

REMEMBER!

The layers or strata of the epidermis have different names depending on what textbook you refer to. There is a simple rhyme you should remember to give you a correct version of the layers.

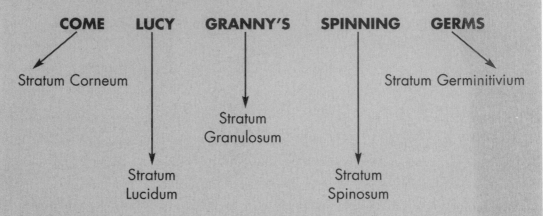

| COME | LUCY | GRANNY'S | SPINNING | GERMS |

Stratum Corneum

Stratum Granulosum

Stratum Lucidum

Stratum Spinosum

Stratum Germinitivium

The stratum corneum is the uppermost layer, and the stratum germinitivum is the bottom layer.

Review your course notes to gain information about the different cell layers.

The Dermis

Make sure you know what structures are found in the dermis. *Remember*, the dermis is a very important layer. You should also know about the papillary layer and the reticular layer.

The Subcutaneous Layer

This layer is sometimes called the subcutis or the hypodermis. Make sure you know some features of this layer. *Remember*, this layer is below the Dermis. Refer to the Revision Maps around skin structure and skin function.

In preparation for assessments, review your course notes and practise drawing freehand the diagram of the skin so that you know it off by heart. When you are ready, attempt Task 1.

Revision Map – Skin Structure
The Epidermis, Dermis and Subcutis

Remember the Rhyme 'Come Lucy Granny's Spinning Germs'

Epidermis has five layers or strata:
1. Uppermost strata is the *Stratum Corneum* – scaly, dead close flat cells.
2. *Stratum Lucidum* – clear, no nuclei, cells bathed in fatty substance eledir.
3. *Stratum Granulosum* – cells harden and change here through keratinization.
4. *Stratum Spinosum* – prickly cells in layers. Lower levels can divide. Upper levels begin to keratinize.
5. *Stratum Germinitivum* – reproducing layer attached to dermis at lower levels. Receives nutrients, mitosis occurs. Melanin-producing cells (melanin affects skin colour).

The Subcutis
Thick layer of connective tissue
- Help keeps body warm.
- Contains adipose tissue to cushion blows.
- Contains areolar tissue to aid flexibility.
- Contains major arteries and veins.
- Contains nerve endings.

Dermis contains:
- Nerves.
- Blood and lymph capillaries.
- Arrector pili muscles.
- Sweat and sebaceous glands.
- It has high water content.

Dermis has two layers:
1. Upper superficial papillary layer.
2. Lower, deep reticular layer, tough and fibrous.

Revision Map – Skin Structure
Appendages of the Skin and their Functions

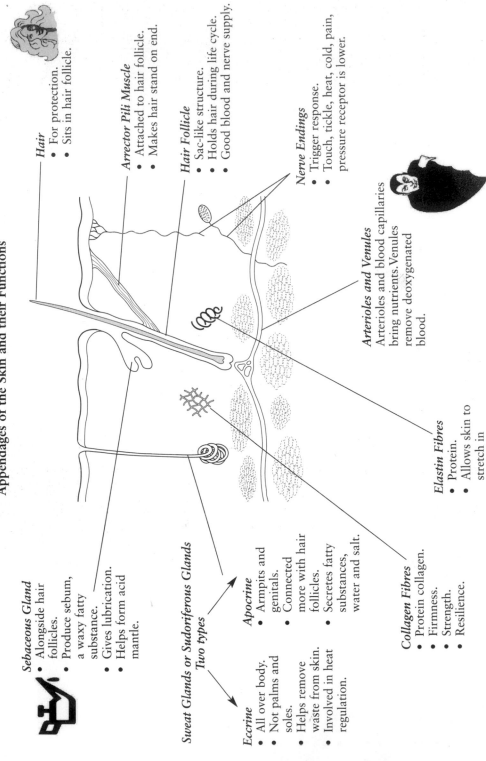

Hair
- For protection.
- Sits in hair follicle.

Arrector Pili Muscle
- Attached to hair follicle.
- Makes hair stand on end.

Hair Follicle
- Sac-like structure.
- Holds hair during life cycle.
- Good blood and nerve supply.

Nerve Endings
- Trigger response.
- Touch, tickle, heat, cold, pain, pressure receptor is lower.

Arterioles and Venules
Arterioles and blood capillaries bring nutrients. Venules remove deoxygenated blood.

Elastin Fibres
- Protein.
- Allows skin to stretch in

Collagen Fibres
- Protein collagen.
- Firmness.
- Strength.
- Resilience.

Apocrine
- Armpits and genitals.
- Connected more with hair follicles.
- Secretes fatty substances, water and salt.

Eccrine
- All over body.
- Not palms and soles.
- Helps remove waste from skin.
- Involved in heat regulation.

Sweat Glands or Sudoriferous Glands
Two types

Sebaceous Gland
- Alongside hair follicles.
- Produce sebum, a waxy fatty substance.
- Gives lubrication.
- Helps form acid mantle.

TASK 1　Label the diagram below – the structure of the skin

(Don't be put off if the diagram is different to the one you are used to. Take your time, do it step by step.)

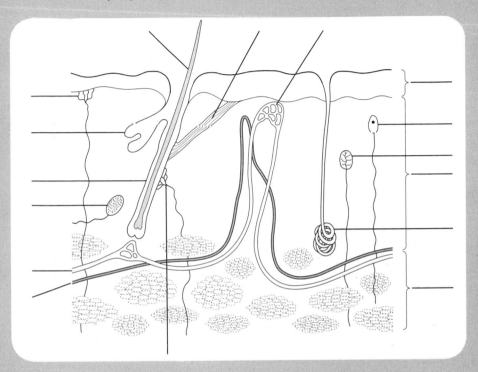

All correct　　　　　　Excellent, well done

One or two errors　　　Well done, make sure you know where you went wrong

Many errors　　　　　　Don't panic. Go back to your course notes, go through the text on drawing the skin and then have another go

THE FUNCTIONS OF THE SKIN

The skin has many functions vital to health and life. To prompt your revision, remember the word **shape**. You will then have the first letter of the main functions of the skin.

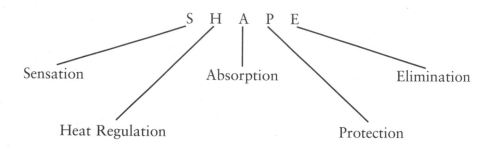

S H A P E

Sensation   Absorption   Elimination

Heat Regulation   Protection

Study the Revision Map to expand on the main functions.

SHORT ANSWER QUESTIONS

An example of some model questions and answers around skin structure and function are provided for you. Reading through the samples will help give you an insight on how to answer questions properly and will also help your revision process.

Q1. Describe the subcutis. *(5 marks)*

Answer: The subcutis is a deep layer of connective tissue found below the dermis. The subcutis contains adipose tissue which cushions the underlying structures from external blows and acts as an insulator. It also contains areolar tissue which assists the flexibility of this layer. Housed in the subcutis are nerve endings, collagen and elastin fibres and blood and lymph vessels.

Q2. What is melanin and where is it produced? *(3 marks)*

Answer: Melanin is the pigment which gives the skin its colour. It is produced by cells called melanocytes, which are found in the deepest layer of the epidermis known as the stratum germinitivum.

Q3. Describe the stratum corneum. *(3 marks)*

Revision Map – The Functions of the Skin

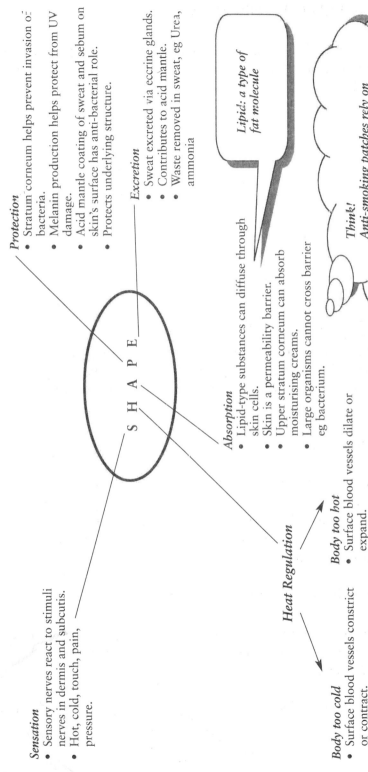

Sensation

- Sensory nerves react to stimuli nerves in dermis and subcutis.
- Hot, cold, touch, pain, pressure.

Protection

- Stratum corneum helps prevent invasion of bacteria.
- Melanin production helps protect from UV damage.
- Acid mantle coating of sweat and sebum on skin's surface has anti-bacterial role.
- Protects underlying structure.

Excretion

- Sweat excreted via eccrine glands.
- Contributes to acid mantle.
- Waste removed in sweat, eg Urea, ammonia

Lipid: a type of fat molecule

Think!
Anti-smoking patches rely on absorption though diffusion.
Some cosmetic preparations contain ingredients that are also absorbed by diffusion

Absorption

- Lipid-type substances can diffuse through skin cells.
- Skin is a permeability barrier.
- Upper stratum corneum can absorb moisturising creams.
- Large organisms cannot cross barrier eg bacterium.

SHAPE

Heat Regulation

Body too hot

- Surface blood vessels dilate or expand.
- Extra blood at skin's surface.
- Cooling assisted by convection, conduction, radiation.
- Correct name 'Vasodilation'.
- Sudoriferous glands produce sweat.
- Helps cool the body.

Body too cold

- Surface blood vessels constrict or contract.
- Less blood at skin's surface.
- Blood kept around deeper organs.
- Correct name 'Vasoconstriction'.
- Arrector pili muscles contract.
- Hair stands on end.
- Air trapped close to body.

Answer: The stratum corneum is the uppermost layer of the epidermis. The stratum corneum consists of many layers of tough, horny, keratinized cells which are tightly packed together. The cells are dead, have no nuclei and are constantly being shed and replaced.

Q4. What is keratinization? In which cell layer of the epidermis does keratinization begin? *(4 marks)*

Answer: Keratinization is the process through which living cells containing a nucleus change into flat, dead, keratin filled cells, without a nucleus. Keratinization begins through chemical changes in the upper part of the stratum spinosum.

Q5. Compare the reticular layer of the dermis to the papillary layer of the dermis. *(10 marks)*

Answer: The reticular layer is the deeper layer. It is made up of tough connective tissue. It contains an intricate network of fine veins, small arteries, lymph vessels and many sensory nerve endings. Also present are collagen and elastin fibres, which contribute to skin tone and appearance. The hair follicle, sebaceous gland, arrector pili muscle and sweat glands are frequently found settled in this deeper, stronger layer.

The papillary layer is the more superficial layer. It contains some nerve endings and has a fine capillary network, which contributes to the nourishment of the lower epidermal layers. This layer is composed of adipose connective tissue which is not as dense as the connective tissues of the reticular layer. The papillary layer is connected to the epidermis by a series of protrusions called dermal papillae. The dermal papillae can be profound enough to give the overlying epidermis an uneven appearance.

Q6. Where is the arrector pili muscle found, and what is its function? *(4 marks)*

Answer: The arrector pili muscle is found in the dermis. It runs from the side of the hair follicle to the lowest point of the epidermis. The arrector pili muscle contracts to raise the hair from the skin's surface. This occurs as part of the heat regulation process or as a response to fear.

Q7. Why is there a concentration of blood capillaries around the hair follicle? *(2 marks)*

Answer: The hair follicle is the sac-like structure which contains the hair during its life cycle. The hair is a living, growing structure and requires nourishment from the circulatory system to sustain healthy development and growth. This is why there is an abundance of blood capillaries around the hair follicle.

Q8. Where are the eccrine glands situated? Outline their appearance. *(2 marks)*

Answer: The eccrine glands are sweat glands situated in the deeper layers of the dermis. These glands consist of a coiled base which is situated in the deeper dermal layers; the coiled base opens into a tube-like structure which ascends through the dermis, then the epidermis, to the skin's surface. The opening is called a sweat pore.

Q9. Where are the apocrine glands found? Briefly outline them. *(2 marks)*

Answer: These glands are found in the genital, underarm and breast areas. They open into hair follicles and produce a thicker secretion than the eccrine glands. There are less apocrine glands than eccrine glands, and they fall under the control of the central nervous system.

Q10. Define the term vasoconstriction. *(2 marks)*

Answer: The term vasoconstriction refers to the contraction or constriction of the peripheral blood vessels in the skin to help retain the body's heat. This is a normal response and is part of the body's heat regulation process.

Q11. When does vasodilation occur? What is vasodilation? *(4 marks)*

Answer: Vasodilation occurs when the body temperature rises. In vasodilation the peripheral blood vessels of the skin dilate, allowing extra blood to be brought to the skin's surface. Excess heat can then be lost through the skin's surface by convection, radiation and conduction.

Q12. In which layer of the epidermis does mitosis occur? *(1 mark)*

Answer: In the stratum germinitivum.

Q13. Outline the position of the sebaceous gland in the skin. What does this gland secrete? *(2 marks)*

Answer: The sebaceous gland is positioned in the dermis. The sebaceous gland opens into the hair follicle. Sebum is secreted by this gland.

Q14. State two functions of Sebum *(2 marks)*

Possible Answers:
- Sebum is produced to lubricate the skin and hair.
- Sebum combines with sweat on the skin's surface to produce the acid mantle of the skin which has a protective role.
- The waxy nature of sebum helps to keep the skin waterproof.

Q15. What are the sensory nerve endings of the skin, and where can they be found?
(2 marks)

Answer: The sensory nerve endings of the skin respond to stimuli such as touch, pain, heat, cold and pressure. They are situated mainly in the dermis and subcutis at varying levels. There are also receptors in the stratum germinitivum.

SKIN TYPES AND COMMON SKIN CONDITIONS

As a beauty therapist you must be able to accurately identify skin types and skin disorders. You should understand their possible causes and, more importantly, know how to improve the appearance and function of the client's skin by the treatments and advice you offer.

 REMEMBER!

Skin conditions can be improved by beauty therapy treatments. Skin conditions are quite different to skin diseases which would generally be contra-indicated to beauty therapy treatments.

Skin types can be defined as:
- oily
- dry
- combination.

Skin conditions can be defined as:
- sensitive
- comedones
- milia
- dehyrated
- broken capillaries
- mature
- seborrhoeic

Refer to your course notes and Revision Maps and then review the model questions and answers provided for you.

Revision Map – Skin Types

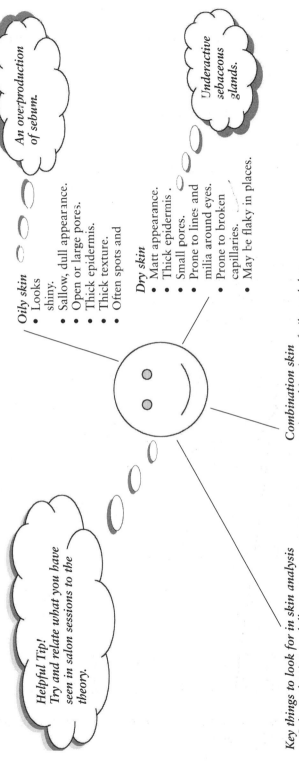

Oily skin
- Looks shiny.
- Sallow, dull appearance.
- Open or large pores.
- Thick epidermis.
- Thick texture.
- Often spots and

An overproduction of sebum.

Dry skin
- Matt appearance.
- Thick epidermis .
- Small pores.
- Prone to lines and milia around eyes.
- Prone to broken capillaries.
- May be flaky in places.

Underactive sebaceous glands.

The T Zone

Combination skin
- A combination of oily and dry characteristics.
- Mainly oily across nose, forehead and chin.
- Dry on cheeks.

Needs to be cared for and treated as two separate skin types.

Key things to look for in skin analysis
- Colour, glowing or dull.
- Texture, fine or coarse.
- Pore size, small or orange peel.
- Tone, firm and elastic or sagging.
- Shiny? Check the T Zone.
- Lines, fine or deep.
- Irregularities, eg scars, moles.
- Broken capillaries.
- Care – does the skin look cared for?

Helpful Tip!
Try and relate what you have seen in salon sessions to the theory.

Revision Map – Skin Conditions

Comedones
- Blackheads.
- Linked with oily skins.
- Sebum under a layer of dead skin cells, darkens when in contact with air.
- Most common on nose and chin.
- Possible cause, too much sebum, not enough exfoliation.

Milia
- Whiteheads.
- Sebum trapped in covered follicle.
- Characteristic of dry skin found around eye area.
- Can feel quite hard.

Dehydrated
- Extremely lacking in moisture.
- Parched fine appearance.
- Prone to fine lines, broken capillaries and sensitivity.
- Possible causes: lack of care, illness, harsh products, working conditions, eg air conditioning.

Broken Capillaries
- Thin walled capillaries near skin's surface rupture.
- Affects cheeks and nose area.
- Common in skins with thin epidermis.
- Possible causes: neglect, harsh treatment, working environment eg outdoors.

Mature Skin
- Heavily lined, crepey.
- Poor underlying muscle tone.
- Poor elasticity and tone (firmness).
- Can appear thin (parchment).
- Colour poor.
- Pigmentation uneven.
- Causes: general ageing process.

Remember, skin will age prematurely if over exposed to the sun.

Seborrhoeic
- Severely overactive glands.
- Extremely oily, shiny.
- Spots and blackheads.
- Difficult to control.
- Thick appearance and texture.
- Sometimes scalp and chest affected.

Sensitive
- Linked more with dry skin types.
- Thin epidermis.
- Easily stimulated.
- Often flaky.
- Small pores.
- Broken capillaries.
- Some possible causes: lifestyle heating, air conditioning use of harsh products hereditary.

Remember, any skin type can be sensitive.

SHORT ANSWER QUESTIONS

An example of some model questions and answers around skin types and skin conditions is provided for you. Reading through the sample will help give you an insight on how to answer questions properly, and will also help your revision process.

Q1. Describe the appearance of an oily skin type. *(3 marks)*

Answer: Oily skin has a shiny appearance, a thick epidermis and open pores. The texture of the skin appears coarse. There may be pustules and comedones present, especially in the central T Zone area. The skin colour may be sallow.

Q2. How does the skin in the central T Zone area of the face differ from the skin on the cheeks? *(4 marks)*

Answer: The skin on the cheeks is often thinner than that in the central T Zone area. There are less sebaceous glands on the cheeks than in the central T Zone. The sebaceous glands in the central T Zone are not only more numerous, they are nearer to the skin's surface.

Q3. What is the main cause of an oily skin type? *(4 marks)*

Answer: An oily skin type is caused by an overproduction of sebum from the sebaceous glands. The sebaceous glands are influenced by the male sex hormones called androgens. Too much of these male sex hormones circulating in the bloodstream will cause an over-secretion from the sebaceous glands.

Q4. Why must the beauty therapist analyse the skin accurately prior to treatment? *(3 marks)*

Answer: By analysing the skin accurately, the therapist can provide the full and correct range of treatments for the client. Proper analysis will provide an insight into the way the skin has been cared for prior to consultation and will also allow appropriate products to be chosen for home and salon use.

Q5. Why should a combination skin be treated as two separate skin types? *(4 marks)*

Answer: A combination skin presents two different skin types, commonly a mixture of an oily T Zone and dry cheeks. These skin types have different treatment and maintenance needs. The use of the wrong products or beauty treatments on either skin type could have a counter-productive effect and would cause a deterioration of the skin.

Q6. What are the features of a sensitive skin condition? *(3 marks)*

Answer: Sensitive skin often has a thin epidermis, broken capillaries on the cheeks, is easily stimulated and frequently has a high colour. Any skin can become sensitive, but skins with a tendency to dryness are prone to this skin condition.

Q7. Describe the characteristics of a mature skin condition. *(2 marks)*

Answer: In mature skin, the ageing process has been long established. The skin lacks tone and elasticity because collagen and elastin fibres will have degenerated. Underlying musculature will be poor, deep lines and even crepeyness will be apparent. The colour of mature skin can be waxy and dull as a result of the slowing down of blood circulation.

Q8. What is a comedone? *(2 marks)*

Answer: A comedone or blackhead is a blockage in the follicle caused by excessive sebum which mixes with dead skin cells at the top of the follicle forming a hard plug. The hard plug at the surface darkens as it becomes exposed to the air.

Q9. What is a seborrhoeic skin and what are the main treatment needs of this skin condition? *(4 marks)*

Answer: Seborrhoeic skin suffers from excessive sebaceous secretion, extreme oiliness and a pronation towards comedones and pustules. The skin condition needs to be controlled with appropriate products that will gently control sebaceous secretion, exfoliate the surface layers and heal spots.

Q10. What are milium, and how may they be treated by the beauty therapist.

Answer: Milium are commonly called whiteheads. They are a characteristic of dry skin, and appear as small, hard, white lumps found around the eye area. They are caused by sebum becoming trapped in a covered follicle. To remove the whitehead the skin's surface may be preheated and then the follicle pierced by a sterile probe. The contents can then be gently eased out. This treatment must be conducted hygienically and with great care.

Note – Regular massage will also help disperse milia. At level III, the indirect high frequency electrical treatment can be used very successfully in the treatment of milia.

MULTIPLE CHOICE QUESTIONS

Some examples of multiple choice examination questions are included for you to enable you to give yourself a short test. Carefully consider the descriptions provided before choosing your answer. Only one answer is correct. Indicate your answer by putting an **X** in the circle: ◯

EXAMPLE QUESTION
The uppermost layer or strata of the epidermis is the

a) Stratum Granulosum   ◯

b) Stratum Germinitivum   ◯

c) Stratum Lucidum   ◯

d) Stratum Corneum   ⊗

The correct answer is **d)**

On completion of the test, check your answers on page 117.

Q1. Keratinisation begins through chemical changes in the

a) stratum germinitivum   ◯

b) stratum spinosum   ◯

c) stratum lucidum   ◯

d) stratum corneum   ◯

Q2. What is the deeper layer of the dermis called?

a) the reticular layer   ◯

b) the hypodermal layer   ◯

c) the papillary layer   ◯

d) the epidermal layer   ◯

Q3. What is melanin?

a) protein ◯

b) pigment ◯

c) muscle ◯

d) nerve ending ◯

Q4. Where is the arrector pili muscle found?

a) alongside the sebaceous gland in the epidermis ◯

b) alongside the hair follicle in the epidermis ◯

c) alongside the hair follicle in the dermis ◯

d) alongside the sebaceous gland in the hypodermis ◯

Q5. Which statement is correct? The eccrine glands are found:

a) in the epidermis and secrete sebum ◯

b) in the underarm region only and secrete sebum ◯

c) in the dermis and secrete sweat ◯

d) in the underarm region only and secrete sweat ◯

Q6. Vasodilation is simply described as:

a) the body's response to a rise in body temperature. The peripheral vessels open allowing blood near the surface of the skin to be cooled ◯

b) the body's nervous response, when sweating increases and the apocrine glands dilate ◯

c) the body's response to an inappropriate cosmetic preparation being used on the skin's surface ◯

d) the body's response to a drop in body temperature. The peripheral vessels reduce in size, helping to maintain blood around the larger body organs ◯

Q7. The secretion from the sebaceous gland is?

a) sebum which is needed to cool the skin ◯

b) sweat which helps to lubricate the skin ◯

c) water which is needed to cool the skin ◯

d) sebum which helps to lubricate the skin ◯

Q8. The characteristics of a dry skin include:

a) thin epidermis, small pores, shiny appearance ◯

b) thick epidermis, small pores, glowing appearance ◯

c) thin epidermis, small pores, tight appearance ◯

d) thick epidermis, large pores, shiny appearance ◯

Q9. The characteristics of an oily skin include:

a) dull appearance and thick epidermis ◯

b) sallow appearance and thin epidermis ◯

c) shiny appearance and tight pores ◯

d) tight appearance and broken capillaries ◯

Q10. The tone and firmness of the skin are directly influenced by:

a) the thickness of the subcutis ◯

b) the collagen and elastin fibres of the dermis ◯

c) the thickness of the epidermis ◯

d) effective melanin production ◯

MULTIPLE CHOICE TEST – ANSWERS

1.	B	6.	A
2.	A	7.	D
3.	B	8.	C
4.	C	9.	A
5.	C	10.	B

Marking and Grading

10 correct   excellent, well done

8 correct   extremely well done

6 correct   ok, but go back to your notes and revision maps and you can improve your score

Under 5   never mind, go back and spend some time revising

SKIN CARE PRODUCTS

This chapter focuses on products which you will need in order to perform cleansing, steaming and exfoliating treatments; ie:
- cleansing products
- toning products
- moisturisers
- exfoliators
- eye make-up remover and eye gels

Refer to the revision maps, your course notes and any information you may have from cosmetic manufacturers.

SKIN CARE ROUTINES

You should also be able to judge how a client's skin care routine (or lack of one) contributes to the client's skin condition. This in turn may reflect on the ageing process of the skin.

Study the Revision Maps and your course notes around this topic, and then have a look at the model question and answers that are provided for you.

The short answer questions also cover exfoliation, skin care products and steaming, and can be found on page 128.

Revision Map – Some Common Features of Cleansing Products

Think!
Why do we cleanse?
- Remove make-up
- Remove dirt
- Remove dead cells

Cleansing Products

Eye Make-up Removers
- Some contain mineral oil.
- Liquid or gel formula most popular.
- pH-balanced or same pH as tears.
- Quickly dissolve eye make-up.
- Contains soothing ingredients eg witchazel, cornflower.

Cleansing Bars
- Contain compressed cleansing cream or soapless cleansers.
- pH balanced.
- Soapless.
- Will not remove make-up.

Cleansing Milks
- For younger skins.
- Fine to remove secretions but not make-up.
- Thin texture.
- More water than oily ingredients – up to 90%.
- May contain detergent element.
- Not suitable for salon use.

Liquifying Cleanser
- For theatrical use.
- Mainly oily ingredients and paraffin wax.
- Melts on skin.
- Looks like petroleum jelly.
- Very hard to remove.

Creams
- Dry skins.
- Nice texture to use.
- More greasy, richer.
- Water in oil solution, eg mineral oil, Safflower oil.
- Oil lifts make-up and dirt.
- Water cools skin.
- Needs careful removal.

General Purpose Emulsions
- Available for most skins.
- A general purpose cleanser.
- Carefully balanced oil in water solution.
- Easy to remove.
- Rinses off.
- Popular for salon use.

Most contain oil, water and a binding agent called an emulsifier

Cleansing Lotions
- Alcohol cetergent base reduces sebum.
- Doesn't remove make-up.
- Not used in the salon.

Revision Maps – Some Common Features of Toning Products

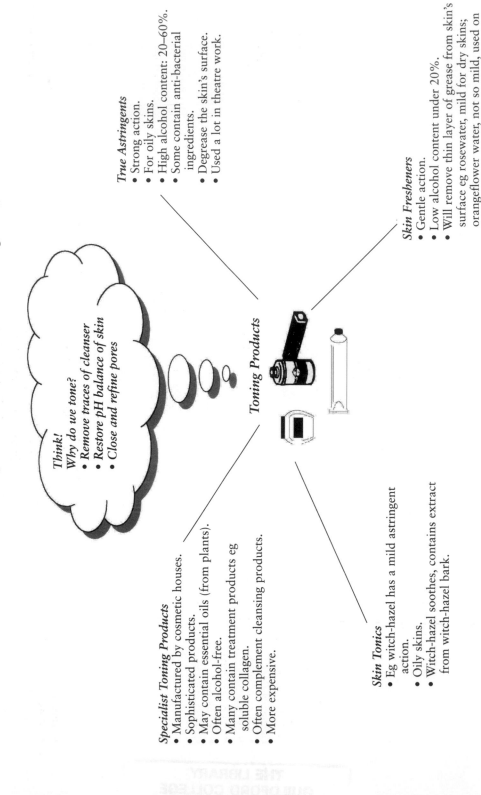

Think!
Why do we tone?
- *Remove traces of cleanser*
- *Restore pH balance of skin*
- *Close and refine pores*

Toning Products

True Astringents
- Strong action.
- For oily skins.
- High alcohol content: 20–60%.
- Some contain anti-bacterial ingredients.
- Degrease the skin's surface.
- Used a lot in theatre work.

Skin Fresheners
- Gentle action.
- Low alcohol content under 20%.
- Will remove thin layer of grease from skin's surface eg rosewater, mild for dry skins; orangeflower water, not so mild, used on younger skins and slightly oily.

Specialist Toning Products
- Manufactured by cosmetic houses.
- Sophisticated products.
- May contain essential oils (from plants).
- Often alcohol-free.
- Many contain treatment products eg soluble collagen.
- Often complement cleansing products.
- More expensive.

Skin Tonics
- Eg witch-hazel has a mild astringent action.
- Oily skins.
- Witch-hazel soothes, contains extract from witch-hazel bark.

Revision Map – Some Common Features of Moisturising Products

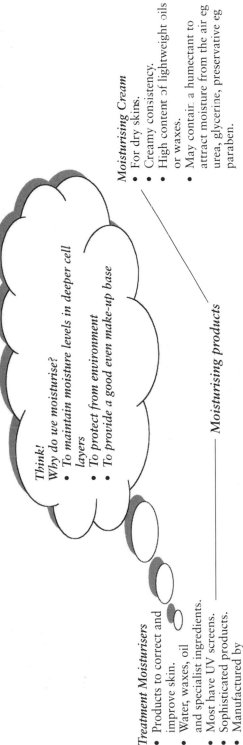

Think!
Why do we moisturise?
- *To maintain moisture levels in deeper cell layers*
- *To protect from environment*
- *To provide a good even make-up base*

Treatment Moisturisers
- Products to correct and improve skin.
- Water, waxes, oil and specialist ingredients.
- Most have UV screens.
- Sophisticated products.
- Manufactured by cosmetic houses.
- Price reflects ingredients.

— *Moisturising products*

Moisturising Cream
- For dry skins.
- Creamy consistency.
- High content of lightweight oils or waxes.
- May contain a humectant to attract moisture from the air eg urea, glycerine, preservative eg paraben.

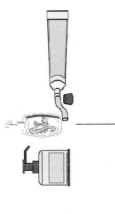

Common ingredients, water, oils, waxes, preservatives, perfume, humectant

Moisturising Lotion
- Lighter consistency than cream.
- High water content 80–90%.
- Lower oil and waxes content.
- May contain a humectant and preservative.

Revision Map – Specialist Products

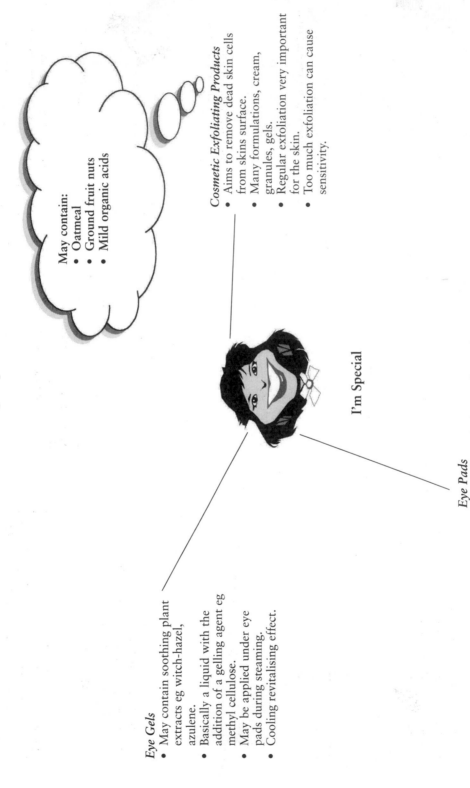

May contain:
- Oatmeal
- Ground fruit nuts
- Mild organic acids

Cosmetic Exfoliating Products
- Aims to remove dead skin cells from skins surface.
- Many formulations, cream, granules, gels.
- Regular exfoliation very important for the skin.
- Too much exfoliation can cause sensitivity.

I'm Special

Eye Pads
- May be soaked in cooling substance eg witch-hazel, rosewater

Eye Gels
- May contain soothing plant extracts eg witch-hazel, azulene.
- Basically a liquid with the addition of a gelling agent eg methyl cellulose.
- May be applied under eye pads during steaming.
- Cooling revitalising effect.

Revision Map – What Causes Ageing of the Skin?

What causes ageing of the skin?

Remember, skin can age prematurely because of
- Neglect
- Ill health
- Sun and environmental damage

Poor muscle tone influences appearance
- Some muscles attach to skin.
- Age and gravity affects tone and function of muscles, sagging occurs.

Stratum corneum thinner
- Gives fragile appearance.
- Less mitosis occurs.

Loss of underlying fat
- Skin less supported – crooped appearance.

Sweat glands less active

Hyaluronic (H) acid in Dermis reduced
- H acid holds and attracts moisture found in areolar tissue.
- Reduction could lead to dehydration of skin.

Changes in hormone production
- Eg menopause.
- Less oestrogen.
- Oestrogen promotes water retention in skin.

Blood circulation slows down so poorer:
- Cell renewal and regeneration, less mitosis, tissue repair, elimination of waste.
- General colour.

Melanocyte production reduced
- Giving lighter skin colour.

Sebaceous Glands
- Reduce in size and secretion.

Collagen production degenerates
- Fibres harden, flexibility reduced, elasticity reduced.

Yellow elastin fibres in dermis change
- Elasticity reduced.

Interesting Fact!
In black skin there are more collagen fibres, so elasticity and youthful appearance may last longer.

Reevision Map – What Indicates a Poor Skin Care Routine

Dry Skin
- Tight, taut appearance.
- Dull and parched appearance.
- Excessive comedones around nose.
- Milia around eye area.
- Flaky patches, flaky all over.
- Many broken capillaries.
- Excessive lines for the client's age.
- Build-up of dead skin layers on surface.
- Feels dry.
- Lacks tone and firmness for the client's age.

Combination Skin
- A combination of both oily and dry skin types.
- Oily area normally T Zone.
- Oily area exceptionally shiny with many comedones and spots.
- Dry areas extra flaky, dry and taut overall, lacklustre.

Oily Skins
- Excessively shiny, greasy surface.
- Dull and sallow.
- Many skin blockages.
- Many open pores.
- Build-up of dead skin layers.
- Pustules.
- Comedones in odd places eg temples, neck.
- Could be dry patches.
- Excessive lines for client's age.
- Generally lacklustre.

Things to look for that could indicate a poor skin care routine

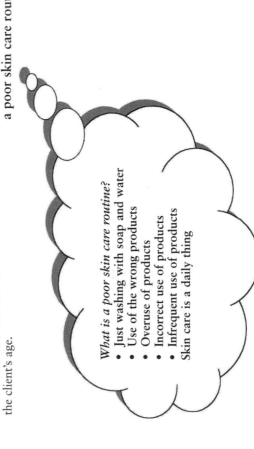

What is a poor skin care routine?
- Just washing with soap and water
- Use of the wrong products
- Overuse of products
- Incorrect use of products
- Infrequent use of products
- Skin care is a daily thing

Professional Tip!
Choose products carefully when treating a client with a poor skin care routine. Products may be too rich for the skin and reactions can easily occur

SKIN WARMING AND EXFOLIATION TREATMENTS

At level 2 we study how valuable skin warming treatments can be across a range of skin types. In beauty therapy, many treatments increase circulation and so warm the skin. This has a beneficial effect on the skin and tissues.

These beneficial effects are detailed for you below. If you learn these effects by heart you will be able to apply this knowledge to many of the treatments you perform (eg facial massage, facial steaming, foot and leg massage).

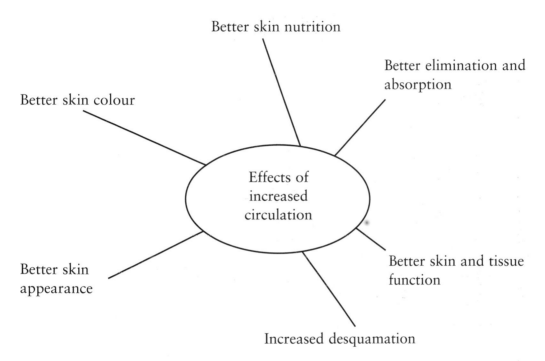

Study the Revision Maps on pages 126–127. Review your course notes and any information from product manufacturers. When you feel you have a good basic knowledge, review the model questions and answers to assist your revision further.

Revision Map – Skin Warming Treatments

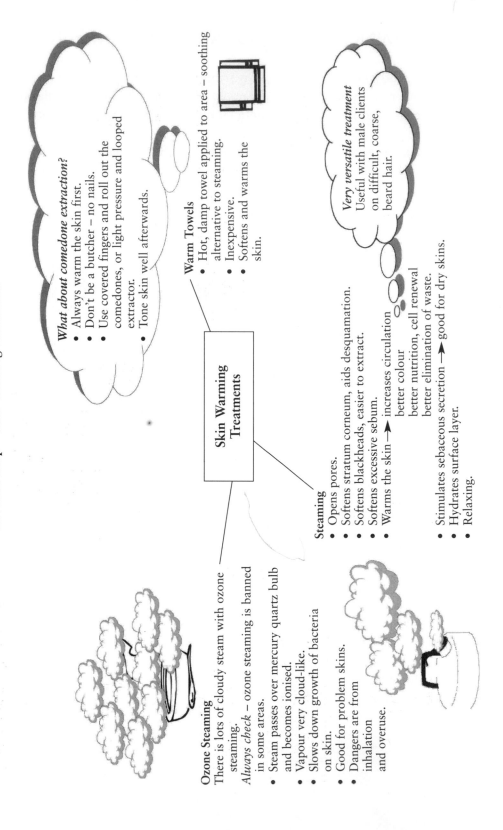

What about comedone extraction?
- Always warm the skin first.
- Don't be a butcher – no nails.
- Use covered fingers and roll out the comedones, or light pressure and looped extractor.
- Tone skin well afterwards.

Warm Towels
- Hot, damp towel applied to area – soothing alternative to steaming.
- Inexpensive.
- Softens and warms the skin.

Skin Warming Treatments

Very versatile treatment
Useful with male clients on difficult, coarse, beard hair.

Steaming
- Opens pores.
- Softens stratum corneum, aids desquamation.
- Softens blackheads, easier to extract.
- Softens excessive sebum.
- Warms the skin → increases circulation
  better colour
  better nutrition, cell renewal
  better elimination of waste.
- Stimulates sebaceous secretion → good for dry skins.
- Hydrates surface layer.
- Relaxing.

Ozone Steaming
There is lots of cloudy steam with ozone steaming.
Always check – ozone steaming is banned in some areas.
- Steam passes over mercury quartz bulb and becomes ionised.
- Vapour very cloud-like.
- Slows down growth of bacteria on skin.
- Good for problem skins.
- Dangers are from inhalation and overuse.

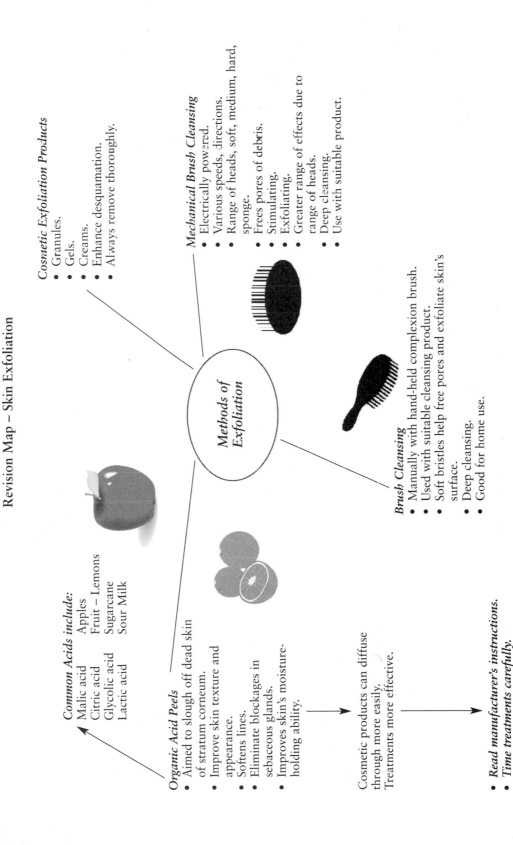

Revision Map – Skin Exfoliation

Methods of Exfoliation

Cosmetic Exfoliation Products
- Granules.
- Gels.
- Creams.
- Enhance desquamation.
- Always remove thoroughly.

Mechanical Brush Cleansing
- Electrically powered.
- Various speeds, directions.
- Range of heads, soft, medium, hard, sponge.
- Frees pores of debris.
- Stimulating.
- Exfoliating.
- Greater range of effects due to range of heads.
- Deep cleansing.
- Use with suitable product.

Brush Cleansing
- Manually with hand-held complexion brush.
- Used with suitable cleansing product.
- Soft bristles help free pores and exfoliate skin's surface.
- Deep cleansing.
- Good for home use.

Common Acids include:
Malic acid   Apples
Citric acid   Fruit – Lemons
Glycolic acid   Sugarcane
Lactic acid   Sour Milk

Organic Acid Peels
- Aimed to slough off dead skin of stratum corneum.
- Improve skin texture and appearance.
- Softens lines.
- Eliminate blockages in sebaceous glands.
- Improves skin's moisture-holding ability.

Cosmetic products can diffuse through more easily.
Treatments more effective.

- *Read manufacturer's instructions.*
- *Time treatments carefully.*

SHORT ANSWER QUESTIONS

An example of some model questions and answers around skin care products, skin ageing, exfoliation and skin warming treatments are provided for you. Reading through the sample will help give you an insight on how to answer questions properly and also help your revision process.

Q1. Give five features of a cleansing product suitable for salon use   *(5 marks)*

Answer:
1. Appropriate working consistency, not too thick or too thin.
2. Removes make-up and skin debris without excessive skin manipulation.
3. Easy to remove.
4. Economical in use.
5. Adequately tested, dermatologically tested.
6. Not too heavily perfumed.
7. Has a retail range to complement the salon range.

Q2. What is a cleansing bar, and what type of skins should use this product?
(3 marks)

Answer: A cleansing bar contains compressed cleansing products in an easy to use form. The cleansing bar is lathered with water and the lather then applied to the skin. Any type of skin can use this product as they are available in different strengths to meet the needs of a range of clients.

Q3. Why should a salon cleansing product be quick and effective in use?
(2 marks)

Answer: The cleansing product should quickly and effectively cleanse the skin without excessive manipulation and over-stimulation. If the skin becomes over-stimulated at this early stage in treatment, further treatment, eg steaming, could be restricted or even contra-indicated.

Q4. What type of skin would benefit from a toning product containing 35% alcohol?   *(1 mark)*

Answer: A very greasy skin.

Q5. What type of product could be termed a dermafloral lotion?   *(1 mark)*

Answer: This is a gentle product containing plant extracts used to tone the skin. It would be unlikely to contain alcohol.

Q6. What is a humectant? Give one example of a humectant. *(2 marks)*

Answer: A humectant (eg urea) is an ingredient often added to moisturising products that will attract moisture from the atmosphere into the skin.

Q7. Why should the skin be moisturised? *(2 marks)*

Answer:
- To provide an even, protective base for make up application.
- To protect the skin from the environment, eg weather, dirt.
- To maintain moisture levels in deeper cell layers.
- To enhance the youthful appearance of the skin.

Q8. What is the difference between exfoliating grains and organic acids in skin exfoliation treatments? *(8 marks)*

Answer: There is a vast difference in the general **application, effects and results** between exfoliating grains and organic acids. Exfoliating grains gently lift off surface dead skin cells of the stratum corneum. This enables better absorption of cosmetic preparations and leaves the skin glowing and fresh in appearance. The grains are often comprised of ground nut kernels or oatmeal, are quite inexpensive and easy for the client to use as part of their home care routine. Organic acids are much more drastic in effect, they slough off dead skin cells lying on the stratum corneum and eliminate blockages of the sebaceous glands. The skin appears greatly refined, and lines and wrinkles can be softened. The origin of organic acids is natural, ie, they are derived from biological sources; eg malic acid from apples, lactic acid from sour milk. Thus there is an increased risk of skin reaction during treatment. Organic acids are more expensive to produce and stabilise for salon and home care use than exfoliating grains. There are also more contra-indications to the use of organic acids.

Q9. Why would mechanical brush cleansing be a good treatment choice for an oily skin? *(4 marks)*

Answer: The mechanical brushing action would deep cleanse the skin, remove dead surface cells and loosen skin blockages. The brushing action would increase circulation which would leave the skin glowing and refreshed in appearance. The mechanical brush cleanser has a range of heads which provide a superficial or more stimulating effect. On an oily skin, a more invigorating head can normally be chosen.

Q10. Why would mechanical brush cleansing be included in a cleansing treatment for a mature skin condition? *(4 marks)*

Answer: Mechanical brush cleansing would be included to gently increase circulation to the skin. This will enhance the elimination and absorption process, and restore some glow and freshness to the mature skin. The desquamation process would also be enhanced, leaving the skin deep cleansed and more able to absorb cosmetic preparations.

Q11. Why is eye gel applied to the eye area during steaming and brush cleansing treatments? *(2 marks)*

Answer: Eye gel is applied underneath the eyepads to soothe, cool and protect the eyes during treatment. As well as the beneficial effects on the eye area this is an ideal way of introducing a new product to the client, which could lead to a potential sale.

Q12. What are the long term benefits of an appropriate skin care routine for an oily skin type? *(2 marks)*

Answer:
- A more controlled skin with less breakouts and a reduction in the shiny appearance.
- Reduction in pore size.
- Fewer comedones.
- Reduction of dead skin cells on the skin's surface.
- A fresher, more glowing complexion.

Q13. How does the client's skin care routine affect the client's skin condition? *(3 marks)*

Answer: The skin care routine undertaken by the client will directly affect the condition of their skin. The wrong skin care could result in:
1. Premature ageing of the skin, early formation of lines and wrinkles and loss of skin tone.
2. A build-up of dead skin layers on the skin's surface, giving a dull lacklustre appearance and preventing absorption of cosmetic preparations.
3. Formation of comedones and milium.
4. The appearance of broken capillaries.
5. The appearance of spots or dry patches.

Q14. What should be used to tone a combination skin following skin cleansing? *(2 marks)*

Answer: Two toning products should be used: an alcohol toner or a stronger product (eg witch-hazel) should be used on the oily areas, and a skin freshener with non or a low alcohol content (eg rosewater) should be used on the dry areas.

Q15. What type of products should be used on a dry, sensitive skin condition? *(1 mark)*

Answer: Hypoallergenic products formulated for a dry skin would be appropriate.

Q16. What factors could influence premature ageing of the skin? *(4 marks)*

Answer:
• Use of incorrect or inappropriate skin care products.
• Illness or general ill health.
• UV exposure.
• Environmental damage eg wind, pollution.
• Poor nutrition.
• Substance abuse eg alcohol or drugs, smoking.
• Taking certain prescribed drugs eg steroids.

Q17. What is the most likely cause of the appearance of jowls and a double chin? *(1 mark)*

Answer: The muscle tone and firmness of youth has been lost or reduced. This would also affect facial contours, and would result in the appearance of jowls and a double chin.

Q18. Briefly outline the differences between vapour steaming and ozone steaming *(5 marks)*

Answer: In ozone steaming the vapour or steam is passed over a mercury quartz bulb where it becomes ionised. The vapour is germicidal and can be used on skins that would benefit from its healing effect. Ozone steaming is not permitted in all regions and this must be checked prior to usage with the local health authority. Vapour steaming is permitted in all regions. In vapour steaming there is no ozone, and effects are achieved by the steam vapour alone.

Q19. What is the correct treatment time for a vapour steaming treatment?

(2 marks)

Answer: There is no specified correct treatment time. The treatment time should be determined by individual skin reaction. The treatment should cease when the skin has a faint pink appearance. Treatment time could be anywhere between 2–15 minutes.

Q20. Why is facial steaming useful as part of a cleansing treatment? *(4 marks)*

Answer: Facial steaming opens the pores and softens surface dead skin cells and sebum. Comedone extraction is easier following application of the warm vapour. The increased circulation will aid elimination of waste and absorption of nutrients, which will promote a clearer, healthier appearance.

Q21. What happens to collagen fibres as the skin ages? *(2 marks)*

Answer: As the skin ages, collagen production degenerates. Collagen fibres harden which results in a reduction of flexibility and tone in the skin.

Q22. Why is the colour of a mature skin condition often sallow? *(2 marks)*

Answer: The blood circulation to the skin is reduced which will directly affect skin nutrition and overall skin colour. In the mature skin, melanocyte production will also be reduced which gives the skin a lighter appearance.

CONTRA-INDICATIONS

Some contra-indications will *prevent* you from carrying out a treatment. This could be because the client is infectious or has a medical condition. Some contra-indications will *restrict* your treatment, eg if the client has a closed graze on the forehead, you could omit this area from treatment.

Study the Revision Maps, your course notes and beauty text books to help yourself become familiar with the various contra-indications you may meet. Some short answer questions and model answers are provided for you at the end of the section.

Revision Map – General Contra-indications to Facial Steaming, Brush Cleansing and Facial Treatments

Contra-indications

Impetigo – Bacterial Infection
- Very contagious.
- Nose and mouth commonly affected.
- Blisters develop which burst, followed by formation of a yellow crust.
- Spreads very quickly.

Extensive or severe eczema

Ringworm – Fungal Infection
- Very contagious.
- The fungi that cause this disease live in keratin.
- Many different types of fungi, some affect nails, scalp or beard.
- Tinea circinata is ringworm of the skin.
- Has a distinct red-ringed appearance that spreads from a red pimple.

Conjunctivitis – Bacterial Infection
- Affects the mucous membrane covering the eye and inner surface of eyelids.
- Contagious.
- Eyes appear red and watery.
- Very common.

Bites or Stings
- Skin reaction could be worsened by products or hand contact.

Diabetic Clients
- Skin is unstable with poor healing capacity.
- GP approval required.

Epileptic Clients
- Most epileptic clients can receive a superficial facial treatment.
- GP approval required.

Skin infection, inflammation or irritation, eg chronic acne

If the client is unwell, eg heavy cold.

Clients with heart conditions or undergoing treatment for blood pressure disorders
- GP approval required.

Psoriasis
- Silvery, scaly and flaky over dull red patches.
- Elbows and knees commonly affected.
- Not contagious.
- Could be worsened by treatments.
- Often develops in 15–30 age group.

Herpes Simplex – Viral Infection
- Affects mostly nose and mouth area.
- Virus lies dormant and is activated by stimuli, eg stress.
- Itchy spot appears then blisters and crusts.
- Spreads very easily

Sunburn

Revision Map – Contra-indications that could Limit or Restrict Facial Treatments

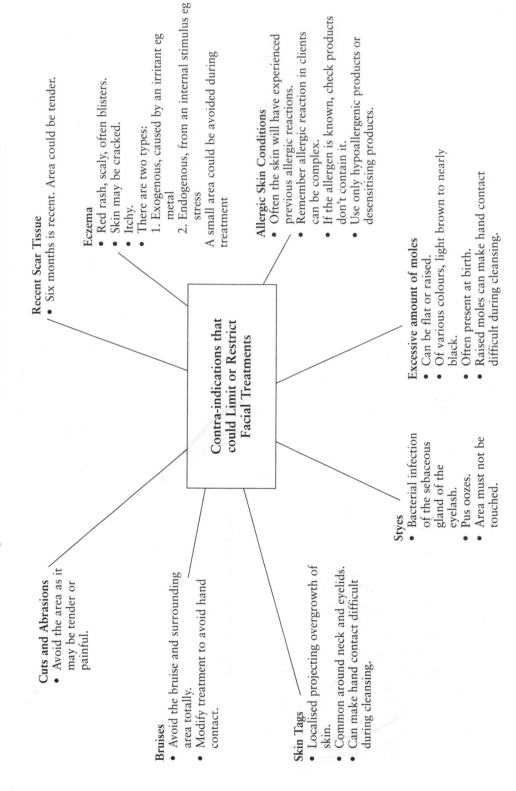

Cuts and Abrasions
- Avoid the area as it may be tender or painful.

Bruises
- Avoid the bruise and surrounding area totally.
- Modify treatment to avoid hand contact.

Skin Tags
- Localised projecting overgrowth of skin.
- Common around neck and eyelids.
- Can make hand contact difficult during cleansing.

Recent Scar Tissue
- Six months is recent. Area could be tender.

Eczema
- Red rash, scaly, often blisters.
- Skin may be cracked.
- Itchy.
- There are two types:
  1. Exogenous, caused by an irritant eg metal
  2. Endogenous, from an internal stimulus eg stress
- A small area could be avoided during treatment

Allergic Skin Conditions
- Often the skin will have experienced previous allergic reactions.
- Remember allergic reaction in clients can be complex.
- If the allergen is known, check products don't contain it.
- Use only hypoallergenic products or desensitising products.

Excessive amount of moles
- Can be flat or raised.
- Of various colours, light brown to nearly black.
- Often present at birth.
- Raised moles can make hand contact difficult during cleansing.

Styes
- Bacterial infection of the sebaceous gland of the eyelash.
- Pus oozes.
- Area must not be touched.

Contra-indications that could Limit or Restrict Facial Treatments

Revision Map – Specific Contra-indication to Steaming and Brush Cleansing

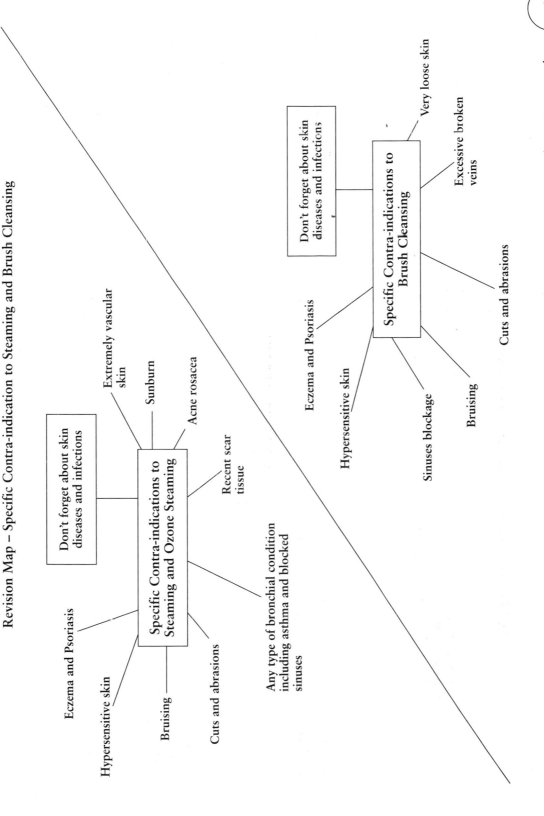

SAFETY PRECAUTIONS

You must know the safety precautions for *all* equipment in use. You will be observed 'working safely' as part of the practical assessment process. Working safely is a major responsibility of the beauty therapist. You won't keep many clients if you give them electric shocks or burns, not to mention broken bones caused through slipping on wet floors!

General Safety Precautions cover the general use, maintenance and storage of equipment. They also include generally maintaining a safe working environment, eg:
- checking of plugs and leads
- maintaining high standards of hygiene
- ensuring any water spillage is removed immediately.

Specific Safety Precautions cover any 'specific care required' when using a particular piece of equipment or giving a particular treatment, eg:
- Making sure there is enough water in the reservoir of a facial steamer
- Making sure you don't get eye make-up remover in the client's eyes
- Making sure you protect the eye area with eye pads during a facial steaming treatment.

Some health and safety legislation is introduced into the Revision Maps for you. Some sample questions and model answers are provided at the end of the section.

SHORT ANSWER QUESTIONS

An example of some model questions and answers on contra-indications and health and safety are provided below. Reading through the samples will help give you an insight on how to answer questions properly, and will also help your revision process.

Q1. **Give two specific contra-indications to ozone vapour steaming.** *(2 marks)*

Answer:
- Asthmatic conditions.
- Any sinus conditions.

Revision Map – Safety Precautions and Health and Safety for the Facial Steamer

Facial Steamer

Check machine for fraying leads or any loose attachments, cracked plugs etc
This is your responsibility under the Electricity at Work Regulations 1990.
The 1990 Electricity at Work Regulations say:
1 Equipment to be tested at least once a year by a proper electrician.
2 This service is to be recorded properly.
3 This is the responsibility of the employer.

Check client is not contra-indicated to treatment.

Position at an appropriate distance for the skin, so that the vapour does not go straight up the client's nose.

Protect the eye area.

Time treatments properly.

Stay with the client throughout.

Only administer ozone steaming if the local authority permits it.

Ensure enough water is in reservoir to perform the treatment
PROBLEM! If the steamer caught fire use the blue powder or black CO2 extinguisher for electrical fires.
QUESTION! Do you know where fire exits are? Are they always open and unobstructed? Does the employer have the extinguishers regularly serviced?
Fire Precautions Act 1971.

Never touch anything electrical with wet hands.

Treat the steamer as **hot**.

Place steamer on a sturdy trolley or stand. Ensure no trailing wires.

Ensure proper ventilation in the treatment room, especially if using ozone
The Workplace Regulations 1992 says the employer must provide certain minimum standards relating to Health and Safety at Work. This includes effective ventilation. The ventilation can be natural or artificial

If the steamer is faulty report this to your supervisor and take it out of use
This is your responsibility under the Electricity at Work Regulations 1990.

Ensure you know how to use the steamer
• If you've never seen it before, get training from your employer.
The Provision and Use of Work Equipment Regulations 1992 says the employer must train new staff in the use of equipment and have all the equipment regularly serviced.

Revision Map – Safety Precautions and Health and Safety for the Mechanical Brush Cleanser

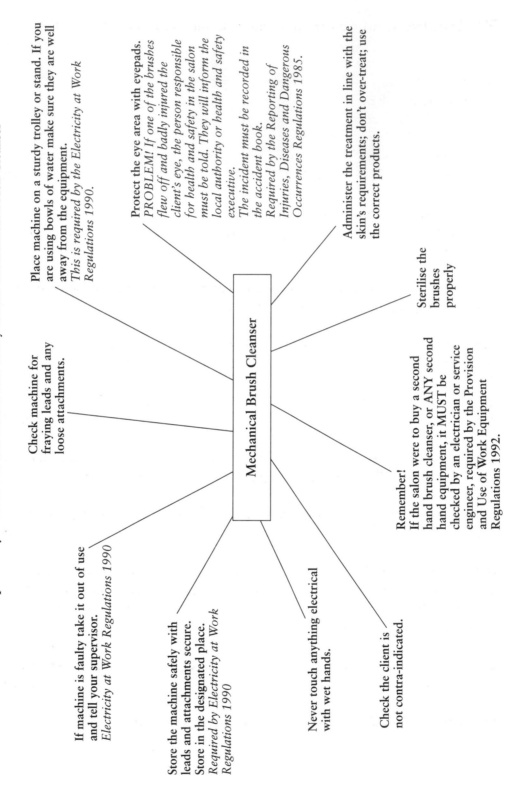

Check machine for fraying leads and any loose attachments.

Place machine on a sturdy trolley or stand. If you are using bowls of water make sure they are well away from the equipment.
This is required by the Electricity at Work Regulations 1990.

Protect the eye area with eyepads.
PROBLEM! If one of the brushes flew off and badly injured the client's eye, the person responsible for health and safety in the salon must be told. They will inform the local authority or health and safety executive.
The incident must be recorded in the accident book.
Required by the Reporting of Injuries, Diseases and Dangerous Occurrences Regulations 1985.

Administer the treatment in line with the skin's requirements; don't over-treat; use the correct products.

Mechanical Brush Cleanser

Sterilise the brushes properly

If machine is faulty take it out of use and tell your supervisor.
Electricity at Work Regulations 1990

Store the machine safely with leads and attachments secure. Store in the designated place.
Required by Electricity at Work Regulations 1990

Never touch anything electrical with wet hands.

Check the client is not contra-indicated.

Remember!
If the salon were to buy a second hand brush cleanser, or ANY second hand equipment, it MUST be checked by an electrician or service engineer, required by the Provision and Use of Work Equipment Regulations 1992.

Q2. State two specific contra-indications to mechanical brush cleansing.

(2 marks)

Answer:
- Extremely loose skin.
- Excessive broken veins.

Q3. Would a client with conjunctivitis be able to receive a facial cleansing treatment and an AHA Mask? Justify your answer. *(2 marks)*

Answer: No, conjunctivitis is a contra-indication to treatment. This condition is caused by a bacterial infection, is highly contagious and would require tactful GP referral by the beauty therapist.

Q4. Why would a client with an area of eczema across the nose and cheeks be advised against a facial steaming treatment? *(2 marks)*

Answer: The warm vapour could increase the amount of inflammatory cells in the area, causing irritation and a general worsening of the condition.

Q5. Why must electrical equipment be placed on an appropriate surface during treatment? *(2 marks)*

Answer: Electrical equipment must be on a sturdy trolley or custom-made stand to avoid any risk of the equipment falling onto the client or onto the floor.

Q6. Why is it important to position electrical equipment properly during treatment? *(4 marks)*

Answer: This is an elementary safety requirement. Equipment should be on a sturdy support, accessible for the operator, without over-reaching which could cause back or shoulder strains. Correct positioning, use and care of equipment is a requirement of health and safety legislation.

Q7. Which Regulations state that all electrical equipment must be serviced regularly? *(1 mark)*

Answer: The Provision and Use of Work Equipment Regulations 1992.

Q8. Which Regulations state that 'written instructions' must be provided in addition to training if required by the employee? *(1 mark)*

Answer: The Provision and Use of Work Equipment Regulations 1992.

Q9. What is the legally required working temperature of the salon after the first hour? *(1 mark)*

Answer: 16°C.

Q10. Which Regulations have taken the place of the Office, Shops and Railway Premises Act 1963? How do the regulations apply to the Beauty Salon? *(3 marks)*

Answer: The Workplace, Health, Safety and Welfare Regulations 1992 have taken the place of most of the Office, Shops and Railway Premises Act 1963.

These regulations apply very much to the beauty salon, and cover the working environment. They provide standards that must be maintained to ensure the salon is a safe and healthy place to work or visit.

Q11. What could happen if the plug socket on the facial steamer was connected to the mains supply with wet hands? *(1 mark)*

Answer: The operator could receive an electric shock.

Q12. What could happen if brush cleansing attachments were not adequately sterilised between clients? *(2 marks)*

Answer: Micro-organisms could pass from client to client, resulting in cross-infection.

Q13. Outline in simple terms the Health and Safety at Work Act 1974? *(5 marks)*

Answer: The Health and Safety at Work Act 1974 is legislation that governs all aspects of health, safety and welfare at work.

The Act clearly identifies the responsibilities of the employer in providing a safe working environment for staff and any persons on the business premises. The Act also identifies the responsibilities of the employee in maintaining this safe working environment.

The Act incorporates different regulations which are very specific and clearly state employers' and employees' duties.

Q14. As a result of EU (European Union) directives six new sets of Regulations were included in the Health and Safety at Work Act. In what year did this occur? *(2 marks)*

Answer: In 1992.

FINAL END TEST

This section consists of statements. Each one may be correct or incorrect. The answer required is simply

Yes or No.

In your assessment of whether the statement is correct or incorrect, you must only base your answer on the information provided.

The questions are arranged in groups in the order that the related topics occurred in the text. After ensuring that all the questions have been answered, check the answers yourself in the back of the book.

1. The sebaceous gland is found in the dermis.

2. The uppermost layer of the epidermis is the stratum corneum.

3. The living layer of the epidermis is the stratum corneum.

4. Melanin is produced by melanocytes.

5. Keratinisation begins in the stratum spinosum.

6. There are some simple sensory nerves in the stratum germinitivum.

7. The suderiferous gland secretes sweat.

8. The sebaceous gland secretes sebum.

9. The sebaceous gland is insensitive to circulating hormones.

10. The layer of skin under the dermis is the epidermis.

11. The arrector pili muscle is found in the epidermis.

12. The accrine glands are found in underarm and genital areas.

13. Oily skin suffers from an oversecretion from the sebaceous glands.

14. Oily skin is not sensitive.

15. A thick epidermis is a characteristic of oily skin.

16. Broken capillaries on the cheeks are characteristic of dry skin.

17. Poor skin colour is *not* a characteristic of a mature skin condition.

18. Collagen does *not* contribute to the tone and firmness of the skin.

19. Elastin is important for heat regulation.

20. Vasoconstriction occurs as a response to extreme cold.

21. The sensory nerves of the skin respond to stimuli such as heat, cold, touch and pressure.

22. Sensory nerves are situated at varying levels, mainly in the dermis and subcutis.

23. A dry skin condition has small pores and a thin epidermis.

24. A dehydrated skin condition could be caused by lack of adequate cosmetic care.

25. UV exposure does *not* affect the skin.

26. A mature skin often has a poor colour, due to its reduced blood supply.

27. A seborrhoeic skin has an extremely oily compacted appearance and is often accompanied by a very oily scalp.

28. Broken capillaries are common in skins with a thin epidermis.

29. Milia is an alternative name for a comedone.

30. Cleansing creams are more suitable for a dry skin as they contain more oil than water.

31. A cleansing bar is merely an expensive soap.

32. A true astringent contains a lot of alcohol.

33. Rosewater is stronger than orangeflower water.

34. Moisturising products are needed by all skin types.

35. Overuse of exfoliating masks or grains could sensitise the skin.

36. Exfoliation is important to remove surface dead skin cells.

37. A poor home care routine would cause the client to develop acne.

38. In the aged skin, both sweat and sebaceous glands are less active.

39. Facial steaming softens blackheads and excess sebum.

40. Hot towels used in skin warming treatments must be washed after each use on a hot wash cycle.

41. The ozone vapour appears the same as normal steam vapour.

42. AHA's are derived from synthetic materials.

43. Organic acid peeling treatments can have the effect of softening lines and improving skin texture and appearance.

44. Mechanical brush cleansing is an excellent treatment to exfoliate the skin and increase circulation.

45. Regular brush cleansing will improve skin texture and colour.

46. The incorrect fuse in a plug could result in the plug becoming hot during use.

47. Electrical equipment should be checked for fraying leads and any loose attachments prior to use.

48. The red fire extinguisher which emits water can be used on *any* type of fire.

49. Health and safety at work is the sole responsibility of the salon owner.

50. Recent scar tissue refers to the scar tissue under six months old.

51. Depending on severity, scar tissue could limit or contra-indicate a facial treatment.

52. Eczema or psoriasis could be worsened by facial steaming.

53. Conjunctivitis is *not* contagious.

54. Ringworm is a fungal infection.

55. Fungal infections are *not* contagious.

56. Impetigo and herpes commonly affect the nose and mouth, and they contra-indicate facials.

57. Systemic conditions refer to contra-indications that affect the body systems, eg diabetes.

FINAL END TEST **ANSWERS**

1. Yes
2. Yes
3. No   The Stratum corneum is dead. The germinitivum layer is classed as the true living layer.
4. Yes
5. Yes
6. Yes
7. Yes
8. Yes
9. No   The sebaceous gland is sensitive to circulating hormones.
10. No   The subcutis layer lies beneath the dermis. The subcutis is composed of connective tissue.
11. No   The arrector pili muscle is in the dermis.
12. Yes
13. Yes
14. No   Any skin can be sensitive.
15. Yes
16. Yes
17. No   A mature skin often has a poor colour due to ineffective blood circulation.
18. No   Collagen does 'support' the skin. Collagen fibres degenerate as the skin ages.
19. No   Elastin has nothing to do with heat regulation.
20. Yes
21. Yes
22. Yes
23. Yes
24. Yes
25. No   UV exposure causes the skin to tan and can age the skin prematurely.
26. Yes
27. Yes
28. Yes

29. No   Milia is commonly called a whitehead.

30. Yes

31. No   A cleansing bar is a soapless cleanser and often is comprised of compact cleansing cream.

32. Yes

33. No   Orangeflower water is stronger than rosewater.

34. Yes

35. Yes.

36. Yes

37. No   A poor home care routine could cause a lacklustre, dull complexion with spots and blackheads. Acne is not caused by inadequate skin care.

38. Yes

39. Yes

40. Yes

41. No   Ozone vapour is cloud-like in appearance.

42. No

43. Yes

44. Yes

45. Yes

46. Yes

47. Yes

48. No   This fire extinguisher is only for materials, eg paper and textiles, wood.

49. No   Health and safety at work is the responsibility of both the employer and employee.

50. Yes

51. Yes

52. Yes

53. No   Conjunctivitis is contagious.

54. Yes

55. No   Untrue, they are contagious.

56. Yes

57. Yes

Marking Guide and Grading

Check your answers and then check them against the guide below. In percentage terms 60% is considered a pass. With this type of end test, because it's a simple Yes or No answer, there is a strong likelihood you could have guessed some of the answers! You should take this into account when determining your grade.

34 correct answers   a pass, well done

46 correct answers   a credit, excellent

Above 51 correct answers is exceptional!

Below 34 correct answers means you need to spend more time revising, so go back to your course notes and Revision Maps, and then have another go.

CHAPTER FOUR

FACIAL MASSAGE AND MASK THERAPY

CHECKLIST ✓ Can You?

	Yes	No	Page No
1. Name and describe the major bones of the skull.			150
2. Name and describe the major muscles of the neck and skull.			155
3. Name and describe the major bones and muscles of the shoulder girdle.			165
4. Outline the blood and lymph circulation of the head and neck.			168
5. Discuss the different massage mediums and specialist products for use during massage treatments.			176
6. Explain the different classifications of massage movements and outline their effects.			178
7. State when the range of massage movements can be used for maximum effect.			179
8. List the contra-indications to massage.			180
9. Outline the long- and short-term benefits of massage.			181
10. Detail the action of the dry mask ingredients.			182
11. Detail the action of the liquid mask ingredients.			185
12. Discuss alternative mask therapy.			186
13. State the contra-indications to mask therapy.			187
14. Combine mask ingredients confidently.			188
15. Answer questions around client scenarios.			203
16. Complete a final end test.			213

RELATED ANATOMY

Learning Anatomy and Physiology can be much more trying than dealing with the most difficult of clients – but patience is the key in both circumstances!

This chapter looks at the anatomy you need to know when performing facial massage and mask treatments, as well as revision points for the practical aspects of the treatments.

The anatomy is introduced first and you are advised to tackle each aspect a little at a time. As a topic is introduced, it is followed by examples of multiple choice and short answer questions and answers. This should assist your revision further, and help you to see if you are ready to move on to the next topic.

Remember that Chapter 3 contains a lot of information about the skin, skin structure, skin types and contra-indications. Information you should know from Chapter 3 will not be repeated in this chapter.

A final end test covering chapter content can be located at the end of this chapter.

MAJOR BONES OF THE SKULL

Examination questions rarely ask you to draw bones freehand, but being asked to label a diagram is quite common.

If asked to label a diagram, never be put off if the diagram looks a little different to the one you are used to. Always take your time, and if unsure of any point, come back to the diagram later. Very often things look a lot clearer when you look at them for a second time.

Examiners like to check whether a student knows the *position* of bones, so you need to learn this aspect as well. Try to ensure you can give a brief description of bones, refer to their *size, shape, any special features*, and of course, *position*.

Revision Map – Major Bones of the Skull

Remember! The skull sits on the top of the spine. Here it is described in two parts: *The Cranium and the Face*

Major bones of the Face

Facial bones give us our facial contours and face shape. They give attachment for facial muscles. Facial muscles help us to eat and have facial expressions.

Zygomatic
- Cheek bone.
- Irregular shape.
- Most prominent.
- Also form part of the eye socket.
- Two in number.

Nasal
- Nose bones.
- Two small bones form the bones of the nose.
- Join with the frontal bone.

Maxillae
- Two bones fused together before birth.
- Largest bone of the face.
- Holds the top teeth.
- Forms part of the roof of the mouth.
- Upper jaw.

Mandible
- Jawbone.
- Large strong bone.
- Only moveable bone of the skull.
- Holds the lower teeth.
- Forms chin and sides of the face.

Major bones of the Cranium

Frontal
- One large bone
- Forms forehead and part of the eye socket

Parietal
- Two large bones.
- Forms the dome of the skull.

Temporal
- Two bones, one on each side of the skull.
- Irregular in shape.
- Found above and around the ears.

Occipital
- One bone forms the back of the skull.
- Has a large opening called the foramen magnus, to allow the spinal cord to pass through.

Remember! There are other internal bones that form part of the skull. These bones are not felt during facial massage and don't affect face shapes. Basically they help form the eyes and nose, and a resting place for the brain.

MULTIPLE CHOICE QUESTIONS

Some examples of multiple choice examination questions are included for you to enable you to give yourself a short test. Carefully consider the descriptions provided before choosing your answer. Only one answer is correct.
Indicate your answer by putting an **X** in the circle: ◯

1. The maxilla is commonly called the:

a) lower jaw ◯

b) cheekbone ◯

c) only moveable bone of the skull ◯

d) upper Jaw ◯

2. Which one of the following best describes the zygomatic bones?

a) irregular-shaped bones that form the cheeks ◯

b) moveable bones that form the lower jaw ◯

c) nones required to hold the teeth ◯

d) strong bones that form the upper jaw ◯

3. The occipital bone is found:

a) in the forehead region ◯

b) at the side of the head ◯

c) at the back of the head ◯

d) at the top of the head ◯

4. The two temporal bones are:

a) irregular bones found above and around the ears ◯

b) situated at the top of the head ◯

c) irregular bones found at the back of the head ◯

d) internal bones that support the brain and help form the roof of the mouth ◯

5. Which of the following statements best describes the parietal bones?

a) two large bones that form the forehead ◯

b) two large bones that form the dome of the skull ◯

c) two irregular bones that form the cheeks ◯

d) two large bones that form the upper jaw ◯

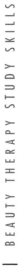

6. Part of the eye socket is formed by:

a) the parietal bone ○

b) the frontal bone ○

c) the mandible ○

d) the occipital bone ○

7. The maxilla is:

a) two small bones which form the nose ○

b) a large, strong, moveable bone ○

c) responsible for holding the upper teeth ○

d) responsible for holding the lower teeth ○

MULTIPLE CHOICE TEST – ANSWERS

1. D
2. A
3. C
4. A
5. B
6. B
7. C

Marking and Grading

6 correct   excellent

4 correct   you're nearly there. Keep revising, review the Revision Maps and have another go.

Below 4   you need to spend more time revising. Look again at your course notes and the Revision Maps, and have another go in a week's time.

SHORT ANSWER QUESTIONS

Q1. Outline the position and give a brief description of the mandible.

(6 marks)

Answer: The mandible or lower jaw forms the chin and the sides of the face. It is a strong large bone that contains the lower teeth. It is the only moveable bone of the skull. The mandible articulates or links up with the temporal bones.

Q2. Where is the occipital bone found? Give one outstanding feature of the occipital bone. *(4 marks)*

Answer: The occipital bone is found at the back of the skull. It has a large opening called the foramen magnus which allows the upper part of the spinal cord to pass through.

Q3. Describe the zygomatic bones. *(4 marks)*

Answer: There are two zygomatic or cheek bones. These bones are prominent and irregular in shape; they form the cheek bones and part of the eye socket.

Q4. Outline the location of the parietal bones. *(2 marks)*

Answer: There are two parietal bones found at the top or dome of the skull.

Q5. Which bones are found above and around the ear? *(1 mark)*

Answer: The temporal bones.

Q6. Name the bones that give an individual their facial contours. *(5 marks)*

Answer:
- mandible
- maxillae
- zygomatic bones
- nasal bones
- frontal bone.

Q7. Detail the facial bones known as the maxillae. *(4 marks)*

Answer: The maxillae or upper jaw bones are large bones which carry the upper teeth and help to form part of the roof of the mouth and other internal structures. The maxillae form a large part of the face and are actually two bones which are fused together before birth.

MAJOR MUSCLES OF THE NECK AND SKULL

Beauty therapists should have a basic knowledge of the underlying structures they are working on. This applies especially to facial massage. On the subject of muscles, it is important that the therapist knows:
- the names of the bones underneath the muscles
- the position of the muscle
- what the muscle does, or its action
- how a person's facial appearance can be affected by the natural ageing process of muscles

A simple and effective way to learn about the muscles is to study a few at a time, gradually working your way either up or down the face and neck, and *not moving* on to a new area until you have successfully learnt the area you are working on.

The Revision Maps introduce the muscles a little at a time. Each Revision Map is immediately followed by some example questions and answers in both multiple choice and short answer style, which should assist you in the revision process.

 REMEMBER!

Don't try to learn about muscles until you feel confident with your knowledge of bones.

Revision Map – Superficial Muscles of the Neck and Lower Face

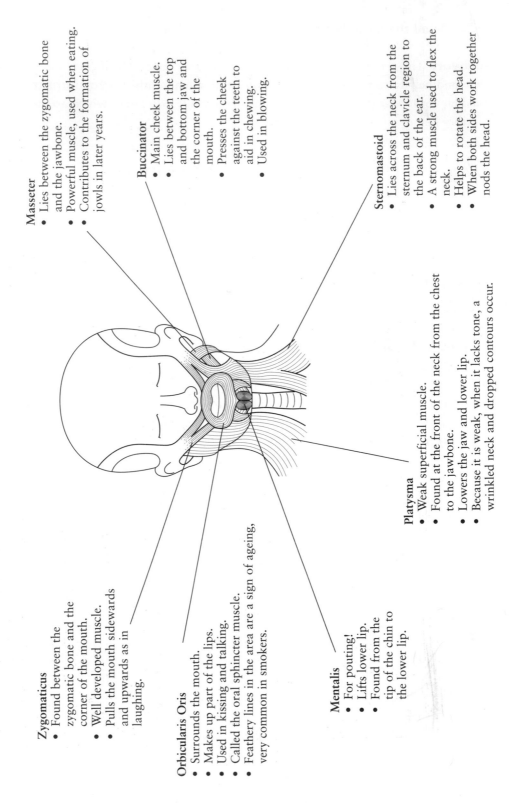

Masseter
- Lies between the zygomatic bone and the jawbone.
- Powerful muscle, used when eating.
- Contributes to the formation of jowls in later years.

Buccinator
- Main cheek muscle.
- Lies between the top and bottom jaw and the corner of the mouth.
- Presses the cheek against the teeth to aid in chewing.
- Used in blowing.

Sternomastoid
- Lies across the neck from the sternum and clavicle region to the back of the ear.
- A strong muscle used to flex the neck.
- Helps to rotate the head.
- When both sides work together nods the head.

Zygomaticus
- Found between the zygomatic bone and the corner of the mouth.
- Well developed muscle.
- Pulls the mouth sidewards and upwards as in laughing.

Orbicularis Oris
- Surrounds the mouth.
- Makes up part of the lips.
- Used in kissing and talking.
- Called the oral sphincter muscle.
- Feathery lines in the area are a sign of ageing, very common in smokers.

Mentalis
- For pouting!
- Lifts lower lip.
- Found from the tip of the chin to the lower lip.

Platysma
- Weak superficial muscle.
- Found at the front of the neck from the chest to the jawbone.
- Lowers the jaw and lower lip.
- Because it is weak, when it lacks tone, a wrinkled neck and dropped contours occur.

Revision Map – Major Muscles of the Face

Remember! The occipito-frontalis is a broad musculo-fibrous sheet that runs from the occiput over the top of the head to the eyebrows.

Frontalis
- The front part of the occipito frontalis.
- Covers the forehead and top of the front part of the head.
- Lifts the eyebrows.
- Lack of tone causes lines on the forehead.

Corrugator
- Small triangular muscle.
- Lies below the inner corners of the eyebrows.
- Draws the eyebrows together in frowning.
- Lack of tone causes deep vertical lines.

Procerus
- Found between the eyebrows.
- A thin muscle.
- Runs upwards from the nasal bones into the skin of the eyebrows and forehead.
- Depresses the thick part of the eyebrows.
- Lack of tone causes horizontal lines over the top of the nose.

Orbicularis Oculi
- The sphincter muscle of the eyelids.
- Surrounds the eye and passes over the upper cheeks and temporal area.
- Closes and winks the eye.
- Lack of tone causes drooped eyelids and crow's feet.

Temporalis
- Found at the sides of the face.
- Strong fan shaped muscle.
- Runs from the temporal bone to the mandible.
- Assists in mastication.
- Lifts the lower jaw.

Levators of the Upper Lip
- Sometimes called the levator quadratus.
- Four small muscles that lift the upper lip.
- Basically run from the maxillae to the upper lip.
- Lack of tone causes naso-labial folds.

Depressors of the lower lip
- Sometimes called the depressor quadratus.
- Four small muscles that draw the lower lip down.
- Basically run from the mandible to the lower lip.
- Lack of tone contributes to jowls.
- The depressor anguli-oris is triangular in shape, and sometimes called the triangularis.
- The triangularis runs from the mandible to the corner of the mouth.
- Pulls down the corner of the mouth.
- Lack of tone contributes to jowls.

MULTIPLE CHOICE QUESTIONS

Some examples of multiple choice examination questions are included for you to enable you to give yourself a short test. Carefully consider the descriptions provided before choosing your answer. Only one answer is correct.
Indicate your answer by putting an **X** in the circle: ◯

Q1. The occipito-frontalis is best described as:

a) a large continuous muscle running from the eyebrows to the
   occiput ◯

b) a large continuous muscle running from the occiput to the
   eyebrows ◯

c) a broad musclo-fibrous sheet that runs from the occiput to the
   eyebrow region ◯

d) two muscles that cover the top of the cranium ◯

Q2. The action of the frontalis is to:

a) lift the eyebrows ◯

b) blink the eyes ◯

c) draw the eyebrows together ◯

d) depress the eyebrows ◯

Q3. The orbicularis oculi:

a) is a long thin muscle. ◯

b) is a sphincter muscle ◯

c) is the muscle that surrounds the mouth ◯

d) raises the eyebrows ◯

Q4. The levator labii muscles are situated from the:

a) mandible to the lower lip ◯

b) lower lip to the mandible ◯

c) maxillae to the upper lip ◯

d) zygomatic bone to the upper lip ◯

Q5. Lack of tone in the levator quadratus contributes to the appearance of:

a) a double chin ○

b) jowls ○

c) feathering lines around the mouth ○

d) naso labial folds ○

Q6. Which of the following are triangular in shape:

a) the procerus and frontalis ○

b) the triangularis and corrugator ○

c) the orbicularis oculi and triangularis ○

d) the corrugator and procerus ○

Q7. The action of the orbicularis oculi is to:

a) draw back the eyebrows as in surprise ○

b) close the eye ○

c) close the mouth ○

d) draw the eyebrows together as in frowning ○

Q8. The depressors labii are found between:

a) the maxilla and lower lip ○

b) the maxilla and mandible and the corner of the mouth ○

c) the eyes ○

d) the mandible and the skin of the lower lip ○

Q9. The temporalis is a muscle:

a) of expression ○

b) of mastication ○

c) which provides facial contours ○

d) which is weak and superficial ○

Revision Map – Bones of the Shoulder Girdle

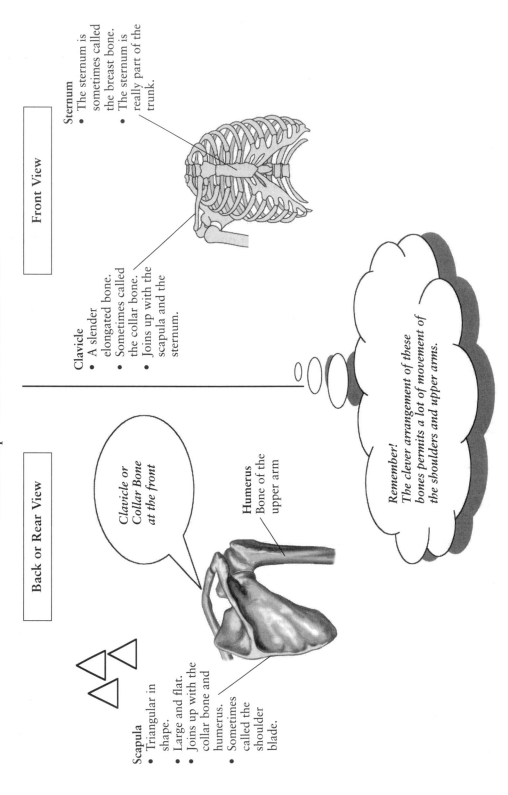

Front View

Sternum
- The sternum is sometimes called the breast bone.
- The sternum is really part of the trunk.

Clavicle
- A slender elongated bone.
- Sometimes called the collar bone.
- Joins up with the scapula and the sternum.

Back or Rear View

Scapula
- Triangular in shape.
- Large and flat.
- Joins up with the collar bone and humerus.
- Sometimes called the shoulder blade.

Clavicle or Collar Bone at the front

Humerus
Bone of the upper arm

Remember!
The clever arrangement of these bones permits a lot of movement of the shoulders and upper arms.

MULTIPLE CHOICE QUESTIONS

Some examples of multiple choice examination questions are included for you to enable you to give yourself a short test. Carefully consider the descriptions provided before choosing your answer. Only one answer is correct.
Indicate your answer by putting an **X** in the circle: ◯

Q1. Another name for the clavicle is the:

a) shoulder blade ◯

b) breast bone ◯

c) collar bone ◯

d) thorax ◯

Q2. The term posterior means at the:

a) middle of the body ◯

b) side of the body ◯

c) rear of the body ◯

d) front of the body ◯

Q3. The shoulder blade is sometimes referred to as the:

a) breast bone ◯

b) scapula ◯

c) clavicle ◯

d) collar bone ◯

Q4. Anatomically, the sternum is really part of the:

a) trunk ◯

b) spinal column ◯

c) shoulder girdle ◯

d) neck ◯

Q5. The collar bone is:

a) an elongated slender bone ◯

b) a thick dense bone ◯

c) triangular and flat in appearance ◯

d) found at the back of the body ◯

1. **C**
2. **C**
3. **B**
4. **A**
5. **A**

Marking and Grading

5 correct   a credit, excellent

Below 2   you need to spend more time revising. Look again at your course notes and the Revision Maps, and have another go in a week's time

SHORT ANSWER QUESTIONS

Q1. Where are the scapulae (scapulas) situated?   *(2 marks)*

Answer: These bones are part of the shoulder girdle. They are situated at the back of the body in the shoulder region.

Q2. Give an alternative name for the scapulae.   *(1 mark)*

Answer: These bones are sometimes called the shoulder blades.

Q3. Give a description of the scapulae.   *(6 marks)*

Answer: The scapulae are two bones situated at the back of the upper body. They form part of the shoulder girdle. They are flat, triangular-shaped bones, sometimes referred to as the shoulder blades. They articulate or join up with the collar bone and humerus, thus providing a lot of movement for the shoulder region.

Q4. Outline the location of the clavicles.   *(3 marks)*

Answer: There are two clavicles or collar bones. They are situated at the front of the upper body around shoulder level. They articulate or link up with the sternum and the scapula.

Revision Map – Muscles of the Shoulder Girdle

Front View

Pectoralis major

- A large, strong, fan-shaped triangular muscle.
- Covers the front of the chest.
- Runs from the clavicle and middle of the body to the upper arm bone.
- Helps to move the arm forwards, as in throwing.

Deltoid

- Imagine a large shoulder pad and you can place the deltoid.
- Gives shape to the shoulder.
- Runs roughly from the scapula and outer part of the clavicle *over the shoulder joint* to the upper arm.
- Rotates the arm.
- Lifts and extends the arm.

Interesting Fact!
The pectoralis muscles or pectorals lie underneath the breasts. The breasts are attached by connective tissue to the pectorals. Unfortunately lack of tone in these muscles contributes to sagging breasts.

Back View

Trapezius

- Large triangular flat muscle.
- Covers the upper back and back and sides of the neck.
- Runs from the middle of the body outwards to the scapula and outer part of the clavicle.
- Lifts or shrugs the shoulders.

Interesting Fact!
The trapezius is an anti-gravity muscle. This means it helps keep the body upright. The trapezius helps keep the scapula in place during some movements.

Q5. Describe the collar bones. *(5 marks)*

Answer: The collar bones or clavicles are slender, elongated bones found at the front or anterior of the body at around shoulder level. These bones articulate or join up with the scapulae at the back and sternum at the front of the body. The clever arrangement of these bones contribute to a range of movement of the shoulders and upper body.

SHORT ANSWER QUESTIONS

Q1. Briefly describe the trapezius muscle. *(4 marks)*

Answer: The trapezius is a large, triangular, flat muscle which covers the upper back and the back and sides of the neck. This muscle lifts the shoulders and keeps the scapula steady during some movements. It runs outwards to the scapula and outer part of the clavicle.

Q2. What is the action of the muscle known as the deltoid? *(2 marks)*

Answer: This muscle is used in rotation of the arm, and in lifting and extension of the arm.

Q3. Outline the position of the pectoral muscles. *(3 marks)*

Answer: The pectoral muscles or pectoralis major muscles are found at the front of the body covering the front of the chest. They run from the middle of the body to the upper arm bone.

Q4. State one action of the pectoralis major. *(1 mark)*

Answer:
• move the arm forwards
• draw the arm across the chest
• inwardly rotate the arm

Q5. Give one action of the trapezius muscle. *(1 mark)*

Answer:
• to keep steady the scapula bones during movements of the upper arms
• assist in rotation movements of the arm
• elevate or shrug the shoulders

MULTIPLE CHOICE QUESTIONS

Some examples of multiple choice examination questions are included for you to enable you to give yourself a short test. Carefully consider the descriptions provided before choosing your answer. Only one answer is correct. Indicate your answer by putting an **X** in the circle: ◯

Answers can be found immediately after the questions.

Q1. The deltoid muscle is situated:
a) at the front of the body ◯
b) at the posterior of the body ◯
c) covering the shoulder area ◯
d) anteriorly covering the upper chest ◯

Q2. Which one of the following best describes the action of the deltoid?
a) draws the arm frontward and backwards, and assists in rotation ◯
b) flexes the neck ◯
c) elevates the shoulders ◯
d) bends the neck sideways and elevates the arm ◯

Q3. The pectoralis major is found in the upper:
a) arm region ◯
b) shoulder region ◯
c) chest region ◯
d) back region ◯

Q4. The trapezius muscle is:
a) a muscle similar in shape to a shoulder pad ◯
b) a strong anterior muscle ◯
c) the muscle that provides attachment for the breasts ◯
d) a triangular flat muscle ◯

Q5. Which muscle runs from the anterior mid-line of the body to the humerus?

a) deltoid ◯

b) pectoralis major ◯

c) trapezius ◯

d) platysma ◯

MULTIPLE CHOICE TEST – ANSWERS

1. C
2. A
3. C
4. D
5. B

Marking and Grading

5 correct   a credit, excellent

Below 2   you need to spend more time revising. Look again at your course notes and the Revision Maps, and have another go in a week's time

---

BLOOD AND LYMPH CIRCULATION OF THE HEAD AND NECK

You should know that massage and other facial treatments like brush cleansing, steaming and hot oil treatments increase circulation to the skin, bringing a whole host of benefits.

For tests and examinations you should have an idea of how the circulatory system works, and should know the names of the main veins and arteries that supply the face.

Revision Maps focus around these points, and a Revision Map is also included around the lymphatic system.

Immediately following the Revision Maps are a series of short answer questions and multiple choice questions.

Revision Map – Basic Blood Supply to the Head and Neck

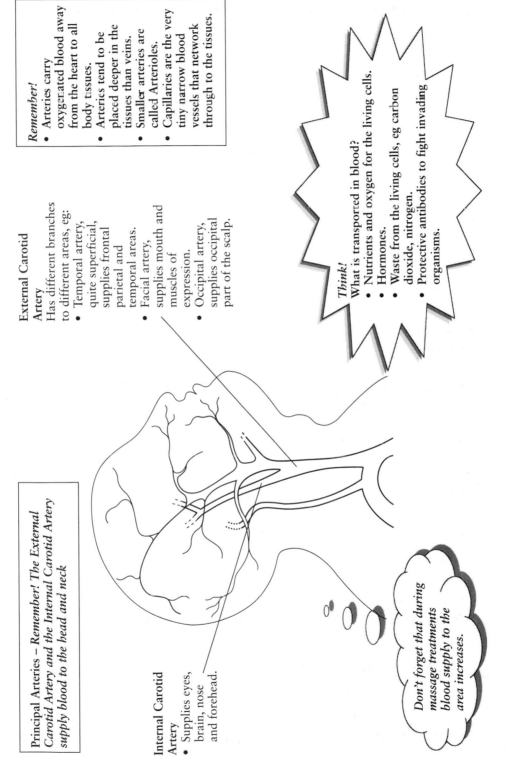

Principal Arteries – Remember! *The External Carotid Artery and the Internal Carotid Artery supply blood to the head and neck*

Internal Carotid Artery
- Supplies eyes, brain, nose and forehead.

External Carotid Artery
Has different branches to different areas, eg:
- Temporal artery, quite superficial, supplies frontal and temporal areas.
- Facial artery, supplies mouth and muscles of expression.
- Occipital artery, supplies occipital part of the scalp.

Remember!
- Arteries carry oxygenated blood away from the heart to all body tissues.
- Arteries tend to be placed deeper in the tissues than veins.
- Smaller arteries are called Arterioles.
- Capillaries are the very tiny narrow blood vessels that network through to the tissues.

Think!
What is transported in blood?
- Nutrients and oxygen for the living cells.
- Hormones.
- Waste from the living cells, eg carbon dioxide, nitrogen.
- Protective antibodies to fight invading organisms.

Don't forget that during massage treatments blood supply to the area increases.

Revision Map – Basic Venous Return of the Head and Neck

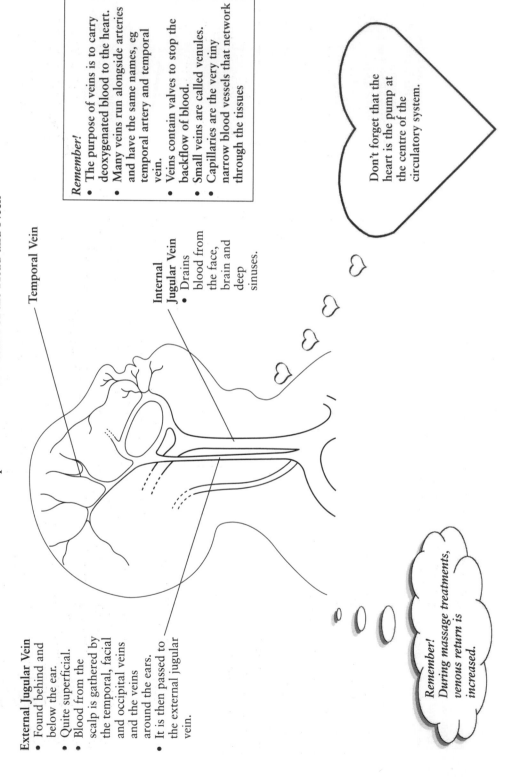

Temporal Vein

Internal Jugular Vein
- Drains blood from the face, brain and deep sinuses.

External Jugular Vein
- Found behind and below the ear.
- Quite superficial.
- Blood from the scalp is gathered by the temporal, facial and occipital veins and the veins around the ears.
- It is then passed to the external jugular vein.

Remember!
- The purpose of veins is to carry deoxygenated blood to the heart.
- Many veins run alongside arteries and have the same names, eg temporal artery and temporal vein.
- Veins contain valves to stop the backflow of blood.
- Small veins are called venules.
- Capillaries are the very tiny narrow blood vessels that network through the tissues

Don't forget that the heart is the pump at the centre of the circulatory system.

Remember! During massage treatments, venous return is increased.

Revision Map – Revision Points on the Lymphatic System

Important Note

Using your course notes or a beauty therapy text book, ensure you know the basic position of the lymph nodes of the head, neck and décolleté.

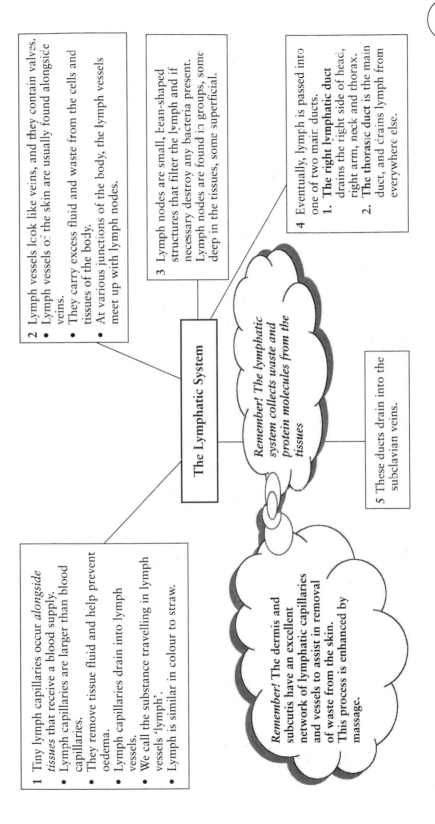

1 Tiny lymph capillaries occur *alongside tissues* that receive a blood supply.
- Lymph capillaries are larger than blood capillaries.
- They remove tissue fluid and help prevent oedema.
- Lymph capillaries drain into lymph vessels.
- We call the substance travelling in lymph vessels 'lymph'.
- Lymph is similar in colour to straw.

2 Lymph vessels look like veins, and they contain valves.
- Lymph vessels of the skin are usually found alongside veins.
- They carry excess fluid and waste from the cells and tissues of the body.
- At various junctions of the body, the lymph vessels meet up with lymph nodes.

3 Lymph nodes are small, bean-shaped structures that filter the lymph and if necessary destroy any bacteria present. Lymph nodes are found in groups, some deep in the tissues, some superficial.

4 Eventually, lymph is passed into one of two main ducts.
  1. **The right lymphatic duct** drains the right side of head, right arm, neck and thorax.
  2. **The thorasic duct** is the main duct, and drains lymph from everywhere else.

5 These ducts drain into the subclavian veins.

The Lymphatic System

Remember! The lymphatic system collects waste and protein molecules from the tissues

Remember! The dermis and subcutis have an excellent network of lymphatic capillaries and vessels to assist in removal of waste from the skin. This process is enhanced by massage.

| FACIAL MASSAGE AND MASK THERAPY

171

SHORT ANSWER QUESTIONS

Q1. Outline the differences between arteries and veins. *(4 marks)*

Answer: Arteries are the vessels that carry *oxygenated* blood, and veins are the vessels that carry *deoxygenated* blood. The structure of these two vessels is quite different. Veins have thinner walls than arteries and their lumen is larger. Veins also contain valves that prevent the backflow of blood. There are no valves in arteries.

Q2. a) What does the term 'narrow lumen' mean? *(2 marks)*
b) Which vessels have a narrow lumen? *(1 mark)*

Answer:
a) The lumen refers to the central space in blood vessels that is available for the passage of blood. A narrow lumen means that this available space is smaller or more narrow.
b) Arteries have a narrow lumen.

Q3. What are arterioles? *(1 mark)*

Answer: Arterioles are small arteries.

Q4. What are blood capillaries and where are they found? *(2 marks)*

Answer: Blood capillaries are tiny narrow blood vessels that form networks throughout the tissues. Capillaries link up the arterioles and venules.

Q5. Outline the main functions of blood. *(4 marks)*

Answer: Blood has a number of functions:
• It transports nutrients and oxygen to the living cells.
• It transports hormones around the body.
• It transports waste materials and protective antibodies.

Q6. Briefly explain the venous return of the head and neck. *(6 marks)*

Answer: The venous return of the head and neck takes place via the deep and superficial veins in this area. Different veins drain different areas, eg the facial vein drains the face, and the occipital vein drains the occipital regions. Deeper veins drain the brain and sinuses. Eventually the external jugular vein will receive blood from the temporal, facial and occipital veins, and the internal jugular vein will receive blood from the internal structures, the brain and the sinuses.

Q7. What is lymph? *(4 marks)*

Answer: Lymph is the straw-coloured liquid which travels in the lymphatic vessels. Lymph is the surplus tissue fluid which is not returned in the venous circulation, but is picked up by the lymph capillaries. It is similar to blood plasma in its composition, and contains lymphocytes, waste products, salts and some proteins.

Q8. Explain the relationship between blood, tissue fluid and lymph. *(18 marks)*
Note for the student
This is a big question, and one you would be more likely to encounter in an anatomy test than a final exam. It is included here because it will help your revision.

Answer: Blood is a type of connective tissue consisting of blood cells, cell fragments and plasma. The cells of the body, organs and tissues require constant nutrition and waste removal, and blood is the medium through which these requirements occur.

Blood is pumped from the heart into large arteries which branch repeatedly into progressively smaller arteries called arterioles, and from arterioles, blood flows into capillaries.

It is here at the capillaries that the exchange of products such as waste or oxygen occurs as the blood leaves the capillaries and enters the tissue spaces (tissue spaces surrounds cells). At this point the blood is no longer called 'blood' but is called 'tissue fluid'. The tissue fluid occupies all extra-cellular spaces outside the blood vessels and bathes the cells, providing the nutrition they need and collecting any waste.

Tissue fluid then needs to re-enter the capillaries to carry waste away. It does this at the venous end of the capillaries, as pressure is lower. These capillaries then flow into venules. Not all the tissue fluid can re-enter the circulation in this way. Remaining tissue fluid enters the lymph capillaries to be carried away from the tissues. It is now called 'lymph', not tissue fluid.

Lymph capillaries join to form lymph vessels. Lymph travels through these vessels. Lymph is filtered at lymph nodes, and eventually returns to major circulation when the lymph vessels enter the thorasic duct or the right lymphatic duct, and then the subclavian veins.

MULTIPLE CHOICE QUESTIONS

Some examples of multiple choice examination questions are included for you to enable you to give yourself a short test. Carefully consider the descriptions provided before choosing your answer. Only one answer is correct.
Indicate your answer by putting an **X** in the circle: ◯

Q1. The external carotid artery supplies blood to:

a) the scapulae ◯

b) the face and head ◯

c) the breast ◯

d) the hand ◯

Q2. What are the lymph nodes situated directly under the jawbone called?

a) parotid glands ◯

b) cervical glands ◯

c) axillary glands ◯

d) submandibular glands ◯

Q3. Which *one* of the following statements is *true*?

a) veins carry deoxygenated blood ◯

b) veins transport lymph ◯

c) veins have a smaller lumen than arteries ◯

d) veins do not contain valves ◯

Q4. Which *one* of the following statements is true? The arteries have:

a) valves to prevent backflow of blood ◯

b) a wide lumen ◯

c) thick muscular walls ◯

d) thin less muscular walls ◯

Q5. Which vein drains blood from the face, brain and sinuses?

a) the internal jugular vein ⃝

b) the temporal vein ⃝

c) the occipital vein ⃝

d) the external jugular vein ⃝

Q6. The right lymphatic duct drains lymph from:

a) the right side of the body ⃝

b) the right side of the head and neck ⃝

c) the right side of the head and neck, right arm and thorax ⃝

d) the right arm, leg, head and thorax ⃝

MULTIPLE CHOICE TEST – ANSWERS

1. **B**
2. **D**
3. **A**
4. **C**
5. **A**
6. **C**

Marking and Grading

5 correct   a credit, excellent

Below 2   you need to spend more time revising. Look again at your course notes and the Revision Maps, and have another go in a week's time

Revision Map – Massage Mediums

General Purpose Massage Oil
- Eg almond, olive, grapeseed oil.
- Feels light – some clients prefer this feeling to a cream.
- Gives slip without being too greasy.
- Easily absorbed.
- General purpose, suitable for all skins and all areas, eg legs and arms.
- Inexpensive.

Specialist Treatment Oils
- Different cosmetic manufacturers produce these oils.
- Pre-blended formulas, eg for oily skin, dehydrated skin.
- Often contain plant extracts, eg geranium, blue orchid.
- More expensive than general massage oils.
- The selected ingredients in the oil add to the effect of the massage treatment.

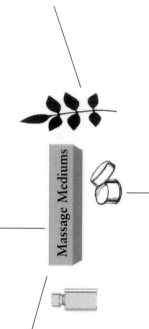

Massage Mediums

Massage Cream
- Various formulations; some light, some richer.
- Basically a lubricating product, often contains a mineral oil.
- Usually a water in oil product.
- General purpose product.
- Traditionally more suitable for a dryer skin.
- Most creams are light; heavy ones can drag the skin.
- Inexpensive.

Talcum Powder
- Sometimes used in body massage on areas like a greasy back.
- Is really an absorbent powder.
- Not used on the face.
- Could be used in a foot massage on someone with sweaty feet.
- Inexpensive.

COSHH – Be careful not to breathe in talcum powder. It can damage the lungs

Remember! Cosmetic manufacturers also manufacture massage creams, again with treatment ingredients. These creams are normally very economical in use and very easy to remove.

Revision Map – Specialist Products for Massage

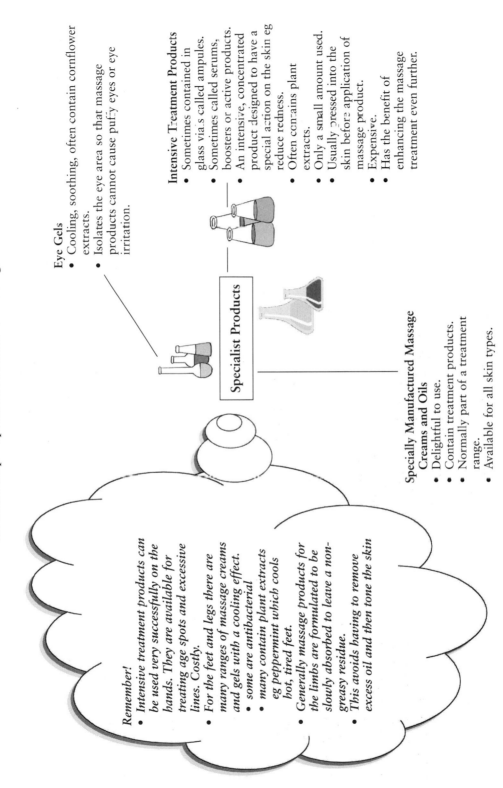

Eye Gels
- Cooling, soothing, often contain cornflower extracts.
- Isolates the eye area so that massage products cannot cause puffy eyes or eye irritation.

Intensive Treatment Products
- Sometimes contained in glass vials called ampules.
- Sometimes called serums, boosters or active products.
- An intensive, concentrated product designed to have a special action on the skin eg reduce redness.
- Often contains plant extracts.
- Only a small amount used.
- Usually pressed into the skin before application of massage product.
- Expensive.
- Has the benefit of enhancing the massage treatment even further.

Specialist Products

Specially Manufactured Massage Creams and Oils
- Delightful to use.
- Contain treatment products.
- Normally part of a treatment range.
- Available for all skin types.

Remember!
- *Intensive treatment products can be used very successfully on the hands. They are available for treating age spots and excessive lines. Costly.*
- *For the feet and legs there are many ranges of massage creams and gels with a cooling effect.*
  - *some are antibacterial*
  - *many contain plant extracts eg peppermint which cools hot, tired feet.*
- *Generally massage products for the limbs are formulated to be slowly absorbed to leave a non-greasy residue.*
- *This avoids having to remove excess oil and then tone the skin*

Revision Map – Classification of Massage Movements

Effleurage or Stroking Movements
- Two types: superficial and deep.
- Superficial links up massage movements, with little effect on circulation.
- Deep prepares the tissues for deeper, more stimulating movements.

Effects include:
- Extremely relaxing, soothing.
- Aids desquamation.
- Aids blood and lymph circulation, warms the skin.
- Improves elimination and absorption.

Petrissage or Compression
- Includes kneading, rolling and knuckling.
- Stimulating.
- Compression movements cause blood and lymph vessels to be filled and emptied.
- Greatly improves blood and lymph circulation.
- Better cell renewal, better skin colour.
- Very desquamative, skins surface freed of dead cellular matter.
- Relaxes larger muscles eg trapezius, calf muscles.
- Improves muscle tone, regular massage helps to firm the contours.

Classification of Massage Movements

Tapotement or Percussion
- Slapping and tapping.
- Brisk intermittent movements.
- Lightly applied.
- Rapid vascular response.
- Rapid interchange of blood and lymph.
- Tones and tightens the skin.

Vibrations
- Always applied with care along path of nerve or nerve centre.
- Little surface stimulation.
- Relieves tiredness.
- Relaxing.
- Stimulates deeper skin layers.

Revision Map – When to use the Range of Massage Movements

When to use Massage Movements

Petrissage
- Excellent movements for increasing circulation.
- Good for dull, lifeless skin and blocked pores.
- Good for lifting and toning the upper arms and improving circulation to the pectorals.
- Excellent for relieving tension nodules in the trapezius (friction circles).
- Small friction circles are good for improving blood and lymph flow to the hands and feet.

Restrict Petrissage on:
- Easily stimulated skin.
- Frail, thin clients.
- Loose skin.
- Broken capillaries.

Effleurage
- Always starts and finishes the massage.
- Useful on tense or thin clients.
- Vital as part of a relaxation massage.
- Useful on a skin that lacks tone, or is a little loose.
- Useful on easily stimulated skin.
- Useful to gently increase circulation.

Tapotement
- Good for firming up a double chin (slapping and tapping).
- Good for awakening a dull complexion.
- Good for skin that lacks tone and is a little loose.
- Omit on extremely thin clients, as it could be painful.
- Do not apply over areas of broken capillaries.

Vibration
- Not all clients like vibration, so always ask.
- Useful as part of a relaxation massage.
- Useful if the skin is very loose and easily stimulated, and thus contra-indicated to deep effleurage and petrissage.

*Remember!
Friction circles can help diminish scar tissue eg acne scars, old scar tissue.*

Revision Map – Contra-indications to Massage

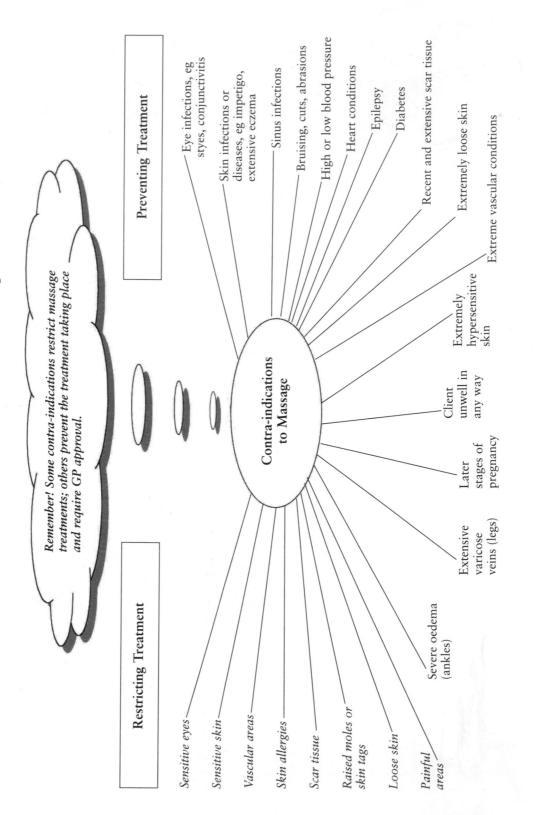

Remember! Some contra-indications restrict massage treatments; others prevent the treatment taking place and require GP approval.

Preventing Treatment

- Eye infections, eg styes, conjunctivitis
- Skin infections or diseases, eg impetigo, extensive eczema
- Sinus infections
- Bruising, cuts, abrasions
- High or low blood pressure
- Heart conditions
- Epilepsy
- Diabetes
- Recent and extensive scar tissue
- Extremely loose skin
- Extreme vascular conditions

Contra-indications to Massage

- Extremely hypersensitive skin
- Client unwell in any way
- Later stages of pregnancy
- Extensive varicose veins (legs)
- Severe oedema (ankles)

Restricting Treatment

- Sensitive eyes
- Sensitive skin
- Vascular areas
- Skin allergies
- Scar tissue
- Raised moles or skin tags
- Loose skin
- Painful areas

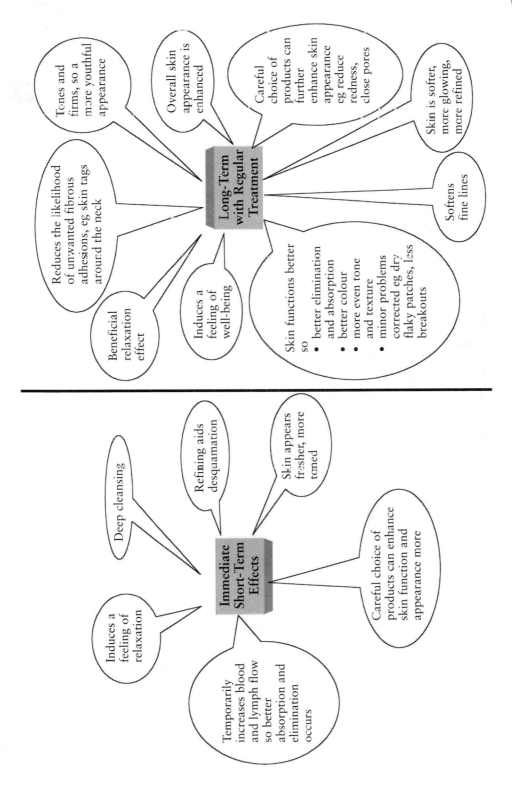

Revision Map – Main Benefits and Effects of Facial Massage

Long-Term with Regular Treatment

- Tones and firms, so a more youthful appearance
- Overall skin appearance is enhanced
- Careful choice of products can further enhance skin appearance eg reduce redness, close pores
- Skin is softer, more glowing, more refined
- Softens fine lines
- Skin functions better so
  - better elimination and absorption
  - better colour
  - more even tone and texture
  - minor problems corrected eg dry flaky patches, less breakouts
- Induces a feeling of well-being
- Beneficial relaxation effect
- Reduces the likelihood of unwanted fibrous adhesions, eg skin tags around the neck

Immediate Short-Term Effects

- Deep cleansing
- Refining aids desquamation
- Skin appears fresher, more toned
- Careful choice of products can enhance skin function and appearance more
- Temporarily increases blood and lymph flow so better absorption and elimination occurs
- Induces a feeling of relaxation

FACIAL MASSAGE

REMEMBER!

Although this chapter is really dedicated to facial massage, the theory of massage is the same when massaging other areas, eg hand and arm, and foot and leg massage.

Being able to provide a quality face, neck and shoulder massage is an excellent way to attract and keep clients. Obviously facial massage is tested in the practical situation, but in end tests and examinations you are expected to know:

- about massage products (or mediums) and their suitability for individual client needs
- about the classification of massage movements
- how to utilise properly the effects of the massage movements
- the contra-indications to massage
- the long- and short-term benefits and effects of massage

The Revision Maps focus around these points. Examples of test questions and treatment scenarios follow the section on mask therapy.

MASK THERAPY

In preparation for written tests and examinations around mask therapy, make sure that you know:

- The actions of the mask ingredients (both liquid and dry ingredients).
- The contra-indications to mask therapy.
- Some combinations of mask ingredients which are suitable to treat different skin types and skin conditions,
- About specialist masks – eg paraffin wax masks, thermal masks.

REMEMBER!

Many training salons and colleges have professional ranges that include excellent products for mask therapy, eg AHA masks, cream, gel or rubber type masks. In external examinations and tests, no brand names are allowed to be mentioned. Testing tends to be centred around the principles of these commercial masks, and around the basic but very effective mask ingredients that we use during training.

The Revision Maps focus around the main revision points, and are followed by some examples of combinations of mask ingredients.

The chapter ends with some examples of client scenario questions, and of course multiple choice and short answer questions which encompass both massage and mask therapy. A final end test completes the chapter.

Combining mask ingredients

When examiners ask you to give a mask combination for a certain skin type or condition, they are really trying to see if you know the *actions* of the mask ingredients. Obviously, it is very difficult to prescribe mask ingredients for a skin type that we can't see or touch; so make sure any recommendations you make are appropriate for the skin condition described.

Look at the sample questions and the model answers, but more importantly, look at the short outline of what the client needs.

REMEMBER!

If asked to detail a suitable mask combination in a theoretical or practical situation, there is likely to be more than one answer that is correct. A good rule of thumb is to think carefully about the action of the mask ingredients, and never prescribe anything that will be too strong.

Revision Map – Dry Mask Ingredients

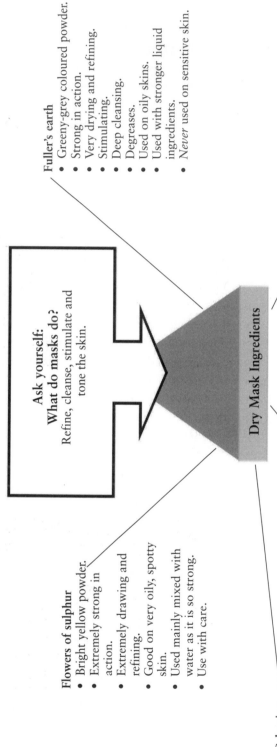

Ask yourself:
What do masks do?
Refine, cleanse, stimulate and tone the skin.

Dry Mask Ingredients

Fuller's earth
- Greeny-grey coloured powder.
- Strong in action.
- Very drying and refining.
- Stimulating.
- Deep cleansing.
- Degreases.
- Used on oily skins.
- Used with stronger liquid ingredients.
- *Never* used on sensitive skin.

Kaolin
- Off-white powder.
- Has the same *type* of action as fuller's earth *but in a much gentler and milder way.*
- Suitable for use on most skin except very dry, sensitive or fine.

Magnesium Carbonate
- Very lightweight, snow white powder.
- Has a mild toning action.
- Useful on dryer, finer skin.
- Mixes well with calamine for use on more delicate skin.
- Used with mild liquid ingredients.
- Magnesium is less expensive so it is often added to mask mixtures to make the treatment more profitable.

Calamine
- Pink powder.
- Soothing.
- Very mild toning action.
- Good for soothing spots.
- Good for calming down a pink skin or high colouring.
- OK for sensitive skin.
- Used with mild liquid ingredients.
- Mixes well with almond oil in a non-setting mask.

Flowers of sulphur
- Bright yellow powder.
- Extremely strong in action.
- Extremely drawing and refining.
- Good on very oily, spotty skin.
- Used mainly mixed with water as it is so strong.
- Use with care.

Revision Map – Liquid Mask Ingredients

Liquid Mask Ingredients

Orangeflower water
- Quite astringent in action.
- Stronger than rosewater but not as strong as witch-hazel.
- Used with stronger dry ingredients.

Rosewater
- Mild toning action.
- Enhances the effect of the dry mask ingredients.
- More appropriate for use in masks for dry skin or more mature skin.

Witch-hazel
- Astringent in action.
- Used with stronger mask ingredients.
- More appropriate for use on oily, problem skin.

Oil
- Mixed with less stimulating ingredients for a moisturising effect.
- Ideal for lined, dryer skin.
- Almond, olive, grapeseed oils popular.

Water
- Distilled water or mineral water.
- Merely acts as a liquid to enable mixing.
- No effect on the skin other than slightly cooling.
- Used with any of the dry ingredients.
- Water added to stronger liquid ingredients dilutes their effect.

Always add the dry powder to the oil, or you will need a bucketful of oil!

Revision Map – Alternative Mask Therapy

Hot Oil Masks

- Warm oil applied to face and neck via a layer of gauze eg almond oil.
- Infrared lamp applied from a *safe* distance.
- Infrared rays enhance absorption of oil.
- Skin colour improved.
- Cellular function increased.
- Local skin temperature increased.
- Good for dry, mature, lined skins.
- Inexpensive.
- Should be considered a treatment mask in its own right.

Paraffin Wax Masks

- Classified as a peel-off mask.
- Always apply over a suitable medium.
- Balances the skin.
- Softens lines and wrinkles.
- Softening, induces perspiration.
- Very desquamative but gentle.
- Never use on claustrophobic clients or sensitive skin or over broken capillaries.
- Excellent for dry, mature skins.
- Working temperature approx 49°C.
- Do not remove until it is cold, for best effect.
- With a course of treatments, real improvements in colour and texture of the skin can be seen.
- Inexpensive.

Peel-off Masks

- These masks form a vacuum or occlusive layer over the skin during use.
- Manufactured masks basically two types:
  - Masks that harden and tighten the contours.
  - Masks that do not harden but dry out, and do not tighten the contours, eg colloid or rubber masks.
- Always follow manufacturer's instructions; some masks must be applied over gauze or special treatment creams.
- Very effective, available for all skin types.
- More expensive than other alternatives.

Alternative Mask Therapy

Manufactured Thermal Masks

- Not for sensitive florid skin or nervous clients.
- Ingredients mainly mineral.
- Special cream applied to the skin.
- Special mask applied over it, which reacts with the cream to produce a warm or thermal effect.
- Generally stimulating and deep cleansing.
- Cellular activity increased.

Biological Masks

- Classified as non-setting masks.
- Often contain active ingredients of fruit, food or vegetable origin, eg strawberries, cucumber, egg yolk.
- Some contain natural AHAs, some are very stimulating,
- Can cause reactions.
- Cellular activity increased by biological masks.

Non-Setting Masks

- May be in gel or cream form.
- Do not dry or harden on the skin.
- Good for claustrophobic clients.
- Often ready prepared.
- Often contain specialised ingredients to treat various skin types and conditions e.g. firming ingredients, absorbing ingredients.

*Note – Vegetable oil mixed with dry ingredients is a typical non-setting mask. Oil is absorbed by the top layers of the skin so very softening in effect.

Revision Map – General Contra-indications to Mask Therapy

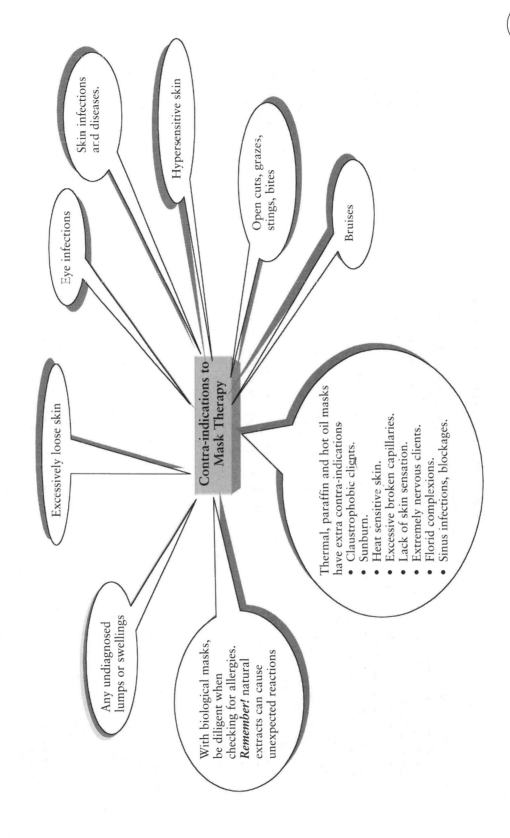

Skin infections and diseases.

Hypersensitive skin

Eye infections

Open cuts, grazes, stings, bites

Bruises

Excessively loose skin

Contra-indications to Mask Therapy

Thermal, paraffin and hot oil masks have extra contra-indications
• Claustrophobic clients.
• Sunburn.
• Heat sensitive skin.
• Excessive broken capillaries.
• Lack of skin sensation.
• Extremely nervous clients.
• Florid complexions.
• Sinus infections, blockages.

Any undiagnosed lumps or swellings

With biological masks, be diligent when checking for allergies. *Remember!* natural extracts can cause unexpected reactions

Sample Treatment Plans

Q1. Give a suitable mask combination for a young client with a greasy T Zone and dry cheeks. She also has a few broken capillaries in the zygomatic regions.

Answer Plan A or B.

Think! What does the client need?

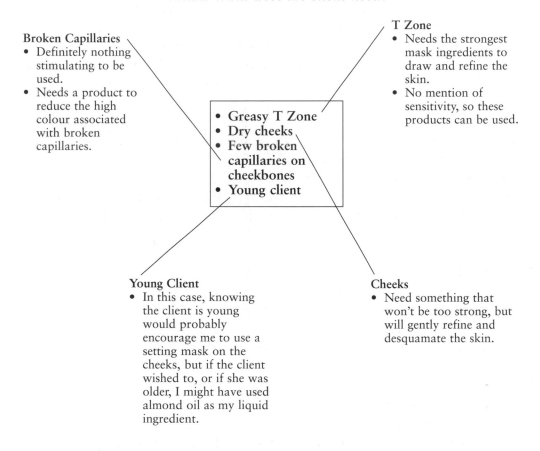

Broken Capillaries
- Definitely nothing stimulating to be used.
- Needs a product to reduce the high colour associated with broken capillaries.

T Zone
- Needs the strongest mask ingredients to draw and refine the skin.
- No mention of sensitivity, so these products can be used.

- Greasy T Zone
- Dry cheeks
- Few broken capillaries on cheekbones
- Young client

Young Client
- In this case, knowing the client is young would probably encourage me to use a setting mask on the cheeks, but if the client wished to, or if she was older, I might have used almond oil as my liquid ingredient.

Cheeks
- Need something that won't be too strong, but will gently refine and desquamate the skin.

PLAN A
For the T Zone
Fuller's earth and witch-hazel.
- Fuller's earth drying and refining. Good for the oily T Zone.
- Witch-hazel good choice of liquid ingredient, will be astringent in action.

For the cheeks
Calamine mixed with rosewater and distilled water.
- Calamine will soothe the redness and be ok to tone and refine the drier skin.
- Rosewater and distilled water as a liquid ingredient will be gentle but effective in action.

PLAN B
For the T Zone
One part fuller's earth, one part kaolin mixed with orangeflower water.
- Fuller's earth – drying and refining.
- Kaolin – also drying and refining but not as strong a fuller's earth. Will combine well with the more refining mask ingredients as it is quite astringent, and will enhance the refining effect required.
- Orangeflower water – ideal for use with the more refining mask ingredients, as it is quite astringent and will enhance the refining effect required.

For the cheeks
One part calamine, one part magnesium mixed with distilled water.
- calamine will soothe the broken capillaries.
- Magnesium will have a gentle toning action.
- Distilled water is a safe choice of liquid ingredient. There will be no extra effect from the liquid ingredient so the mixture won't be too strong.

PLAN C
For the T Zone
One part calamine, one part magnesium mixed with water.
- Calamine is soothing and is not really required.
- Magnesium is mild and toning in action.
- Water – will not do anything for the greasy T Zone.

For the cheeks
Two parts calamine, one part kaolin mixed with witch-hazel.
- Calamine – soothing, ok.
- Kaolin would be fine on the younger dry skin type in this small quantity.
- Witch-hazel – definitely too harsh, it would be much too strong.

Plan C suggests incorrect treatment: The T Zone mask is too weak and the cheek mask too strong.

Look at the following combinations and recommendations; they are all correct and carry a short justification.

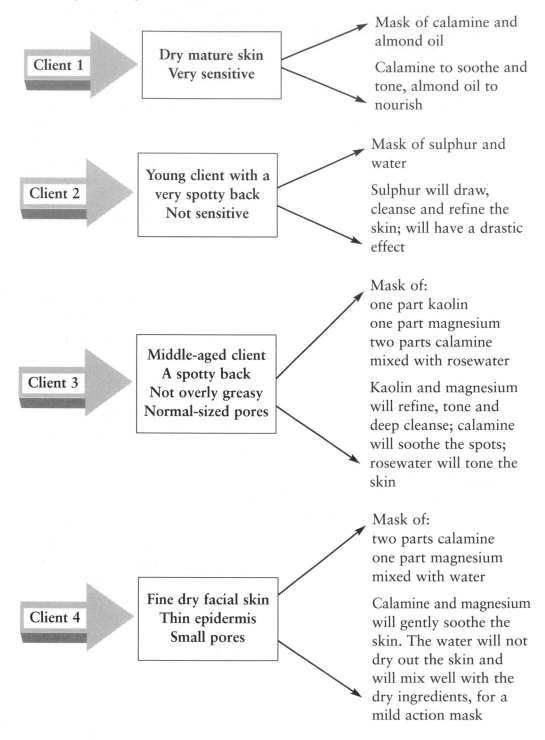

Client 1 → Dry mature skin
Very sensitive
→ Mask of calamine and almond oil

Calamine to soothe and tone, almond oil to nourish

Client 2 → Young client with a very spotty back
Not sensitive
→ Mask of sulphur and water

Sulphur will draw, cleanse and refine the skin; will have a drastic effect

Client 3 → Middle-aged client
A spotty back
Not overly greasy
Normal-sized pores
→ Mask of:
one part kaolin
one part magnesium
two parts calamine
mixed with rosewater

Kaolin and magnesium will refine, tone and deep cleanse; calamine will soothe the spots; rosewater will tone the skin

Client 4 → Fine dry facial skin
Thin epidermis
Small pores
→ Mask of:
two parts calamine
one part magnesium
mixed with water

Calamine and magnesium will gently soothe the skin. The water will not dry out the skin and will mix well with the dry ingredients, for a mild action mask

Client 5 →

Oily, problem facial skin with blackheads and thick epidermis Client aged 25 years Not sensitive

→ Mask of:
two parts fuller's earth
one part calamine
one part kaolin
mixed with
orangeflower water

Fuller's earth and kaolin will deep cleanse, refine and degrease the skin; calamine will soothe the spots; orangeflower water has an astringent action ideal for this oily skin.

Client 6 →

Dry mature skin Lined with age spots, not sensitive Client not nervous

→ Paraffin Wax Mask:
to soften lines, enhance colour, and gently stimulate the skin

OR

Hot Oil Mask:
to achieve the same type of effect

OR

A Thermal Mask:
using a rejuvenating product to soften lines, moisturise and nourish the skin.

Also the client is not sensitive or nervous so is suitable for these masks.

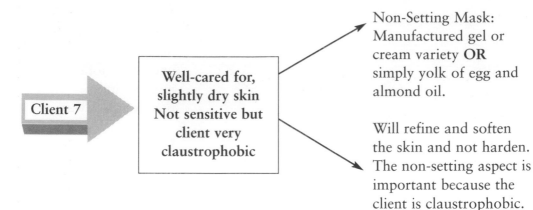

Client 7 → Well-cared for, slightly dry skin Not sensitive but client very claustrophobic

Non-Setting Mask: Manufactured gel or cream variety **OR** simply yolk of egg and almond oil.

Will refine and soften the skin and not harden. The non-setting aspect is important because the client is claustrophobic.

MULTIPLE CHOICE QUESTIONS

Some examples of multiple choice examination questions are included for you to enable you to give yourself a short test. Carefully consider the descriptions provided before choosing your answer. Only one answer is correct.
Indicate your answer by putting an **X** in the circle: ◯

Q1. The action of the dry mask ingredient calamine is mainly:

a) drawing ◯

b) refining ◯

c) soothing ◯

d) stimulating ◯

Q2. During a full facial treatment, a regenerative treatment, ampule would be applied:

a) before exfoliation ◯

b) before the massage routine ◯

c) after the moisturiser ◯

d) after the double cleanse ◯

Q3. Which one of the following is *not* an outright contra-indication to facial massage?

a) skin tags around the neck line ◯

b) conjunctivitis ◯

c) impetigo ◯

d) ringworm ◯

Q4. The best massage medium for a client with an oily, open-pored skin type would be:

a) a nourishing cream ◯

b) a thick oil ◯

c) a light oil ◯

d) talcum powder ◯

Q5. Why does talcum powder come under COSHH regulations?

a) it can damage the lungs if inhaled ◯

b) it is inflammable ◯

c) it is expensive ◯

d) it has a short shelf-life and quickly goes off ◯

Q6. Biological masks are made from:

a) clay ingredients ◯

b) ingredients of animal origin ◯

c) manufactured ingredients ◯

d) natural ingredients from plants and herbs ◯

Q7. Thermal masks are unsuitable for:

a) mature skins ◯

b) florid or couperose skins ◯

c) lined skins ◯

d) dry or combination skins ◯

Q8. The massage movement 'effleurage' is best described as:

a) a stroking movement ◯

b) a brisk intermittent movement ◯

c) a compression movement ◯

d) an alternating movement ◯

Q9. The massage movement termed 'palmar kneading' is a:

a) stroking movement ○

b) compression movement ○

c) percussion movement ○

d) vibration movement ○

Q10. Percussion movements include:

a) running vibrations ○

b) knuckling ○

c) slapping and tapping ○

d) friction circles ○

Q11. Tapotement movements should be restricted:

a) on thin clients ○

b) on large clients ○

c) on double chins ○

d) on clients who want an invigorating treatment ○

Q12. Fuller's earth is used in mask therapy for:

a) its soothing effect ○

b) its mild toning action ○

c) sensitive skins ○

d) to stimulate and refine the skin ○

Q13. The action of magnesium carbonate is:

a) to deep cleanse the skin ○

b) to moisturise the skin ○

c) degreasing and refining ○

d) to gently tone and refine the skin ○

Q14. A suitable non-setting mask for a dry, mature, skin would be:

a) calamine mixed with rosewater ○

b) calamine and magnesium mixed with almond oil ○

c) kaolin and fuller's earth mixed with almond oil ○

d) fuller's earth mixed with the yolk of an egg ○

Q15. The working temperature of paraffin wax is approximately:

a) 29°C   ◯

b) 39°C   ◯

c) 49°C   ◯

d) 59°C   ◯

Q16. Infrared rays are:

a) tanning rays   ◯

b) soothing rays   ◯

c) short wave rays   ◯

d) irritating rays   ◯

MULTIPLE CHOICE TEST – ANSWERS

1.	C	5.	A	9.	B	13.	D
2.	B	6.	D	10.	C	14.	B
3.	A	7.	B	11.	A	15.	C
4.	C	8.	A	12.	D	16.	B

Marking and Grading

14 correct   a credit, excellent

10 correct   a pass, well done

Just below 9   you're nearly there. Keep revising, review the Revision Maps and have another go

Below 5   you need to spend more time revising. Look again at your course notes and the Revision Maps, and have another go in a week's time.

SHORT ANSWER QUESTIONS

Q1. What are the effects of the massage movement known as petrissage?

(2 marks)

Answer: Petrissage is a kneading or compression movement which generally increases circulation to the area being worked upon, thus improving elimination and absorption. Petrissage movements have a toning effect on skin and muscles, and can be extremely relaxing when applied to tense muscles.

Q2. Why are friction circles a particularly suitable massage movement for areas around the joints, as in a hand and arm, or foot and leg massage?

(1 mark)

Answer: Friction circles are compression movements and increase blood and lymph flow which in turn aids diffusion in the area being worked on. This is a particularly suitable massage movement for areas around the joints as it can help alleviate stiffness and reduce oedema, eg in swollen ankles.

Q3. When is superficial effleurage performed in a massage routine? *(2 marks)*

Answer: Superficial effleurage should start and finish any massage routine on any area of the body. It is used to link up massage strokes during a massage routine.

Q4. What type of movement is slapping and tapping? *(2 marks)*

Answer: Slapping and tapping are tapotement movements. They are brisk, intermittent movements applied with care for an extremely stimulating effect.

Q5. Name the muscles found at the back of the lower leg over which tapotement movements are performed.

(1 mark)

Answer: The soleus gastrocnemius or calf muscles.

Q6. What massage movements will help firm and tone a double chin in a facial massage routine?

(2 marks)

Answer: Friction circles or compression to the jawline, followed by tapotement, can be used to firm and tone a double chin.

Q7. Where should vibration movements be performed? *(2 marks)*

Answer: Over the path of a nerve or a nerve centre.

Q8. What massage movements would form the basis of a relaxation massage? *(2 marks)*

Answer: A relaxation massage would utilise both deep and superficial effleurage movements with friction circles on tense muscle fibres. Vibration should also be included, providing it is enjoyed by the client.

Q9. State four psychological effects of massage. *(4 marks)*

Answer:
- Relaxing.
- Induces a feeling of well-being.
- Relieves stress.
- Can improve one's self-esteem and confidence.

Q10. State four physiological effects of facial massage. *(4 marks)*

Answer:
- Increases blood and lymph flow.
- Aids elimination and absorption.
- Relaxes tense muscles, eases fatigued muscles.
- Aids desquamation.
- Improves cell renewal.
- Has a cleansing action on the pores by stimulation of the sweat and sebaceous glands.
- Soothes or stimulates nerve endings.

Q11. Name two contra-indications to facial massage. *(2 marks)*

Answer:
- Skin infections or diseases.
- Eye infections.
- Client unwell in any way.
- Severe sinus conditions.

Q12. State two contra-indications to foot and leg massage. *(2 marks)*

Answer:
- Excessive varicose vein condition.
- Varicose ulcers.
- Excessively swollen ankles.
- Skin diseases.
- Recent fractures or sprains.

Q13. a) Why does a highly vascular condition on the cheeks and nose restrict a massage treatment? *(1 mark)*
b) How should the massage be restricted for this client? *(2 marks)*

Answer:
- This area could be worsened by massage movements.
- The area could be avoided during treatment and the massage routine should avoid highly stimulating movements in general. Friction type movements and excessive hand contact should be avoided in the centre panel of the face. The choice of massage medium must be considered carefully, it should be of a non-stimulating nature.

Q14. How should a facial massage be modified for an extremely thin, frail client? *(4 marks)*

Answer: Pressure must be light and even, care must be taken when working over bony prominences. Stimulating movements like tapotement should be omitted and petrissage movements must *only* be performed over areas of muscle bulk, and then again with extremely light pressure. Overall, effleurage movements would form the major part of this massage routine, carefully applied and combined with vibration to stimulate the deeper skin layers.

Q15. When describing facial massage, what does the term 'even rate and rhythm' mean? *(6 marks)*

Answer:
- *Even rate* – this term denotes that the speed or pace of the massage should be evenly and constantly applied. The movement of the hands over the tissues must not be too quick or too slow, but flowing and constant.

- *Even rhythm* – this term means that the massage application should be rhythmical or harmonious, with both hands working together. Massage movements should not be jerky or quick and then change tempo to slow and soothing. A good massage is evenly paced, flowing and continuous.

Q16. Give four reasons why a client may find fault with a facial massage. *(4 marks)*

Answer:
- The therapist has offensive body odour or bad breath.
- Massage application too heavy or too light.
- Rough or excessive massage.
- Massage routine does not meet the needs of the client or match the treatment plan.
- Excessive massage medium used.
- Massage medium entering the nose, eyes or mouth.
- Massage not flowing.
- Client is greasy following treatment.
- External factors spoil the relaxation part of the treatment, eg client cold or too hot, noisy treatment room.

Q17. What would be a suitable massage medium for an extremely sensitive, dry skin? *(3 marks)*

Answer: Ideally a hypoallergenic massage cream or oil should be used. The product should be suitable for a dry skin and should help correct the dry skin condition, calm down the sensitivity and stabilise the skin.

Q18. Give a suitable mask combination for a client with fine, dry skin. *(2 marks)*

Answer: All below are possible answers:
1 One part magnesium, one part calamine mixed with water.
2 Two parts calamine mixed with water.
3 Yolk of an egg mixed with almond oil.
4 Two parts calamine, 1 part magnesium mixed with almond oil.

Q19. Name one dry mask ingredient *unsuitable* for dry, lined skin. *(1 mark)*

Answer: Fuller's earth (or flowers of sulphur).

Q20. Which one of the dry mask ingredients is sometimes called china clay? *(1 mark)*

Answer: Kaolin.

Q21. Which dry skin mask ingredient is renowned for its soothing effect? *(1 mark)*

Answer: Calamine.

Q22. What are the effects of magnesium carbonate as a mask ingredient? *(4 marks)*

Answer: Magnesium carbonate has a mild toning action on the skin. It tightens the pores, softens fine lines and generally makes the skin appear refreshed. It is slightly desquamative.

Q23. State four effects of a paraffin wax mask. *(4 marks)*

Answer:
- Softens fine lines and wrinkles.
- Balances the skin.
- Gently desquamative.
- Induces perspiration.
- Removes surface blockages and dead cells.
- Regenerates the basal layer of the skin.
- Assists absorption of nutrient products applied under the wax application.

Q24. What type of skins would benefit from a hot oil mask? Justify your answer. *(6 marks)*

Answer: Any skin lacking in moisture would benefit from a hot oil mask treatment. Hot oil masks are especially beneficial for clients with lines and wrinkles, as they appear softer following treatment. This treatment is suitable for a sun-damaged skin or a skin suffering from the effects of the elements, eg after skiing or working outdoors. The warm infrared rays used during treatment enhances the penetration of the treatment oil. The warmth also improves blood and lymph flow, elimination and absorption, so the skin appears fresher and more glowing following treatment. A young client prone to dryness could also receive a hot oil mask treatment as part of an anti-ageing regime.

Q25 Outline the principles behind thermal mask therapy. *(6 marks)*

Answer: Thermal masks provide gentle warmth to the skin without an external heat source. These products are manufactured masks that frequently come in two parts. A cream is first applied to the surface of the skin, and the thermal mask paste is then applied on top. The ingredients of the cream and mask paste react with each other, creating a gentle thermal effect.

During treatment the masks go quite hard and have an immobilising effect on the features. These masks are effective in firming and tightening facial contours, stimulating the skin, improving colour and texture and softening fine lines. They are not suitable for nervous clients or clients with a florid complexion.

In general, the thermal effect must be properly explained to the client. A thermal mask should remain on the skin for the appropriate treatment time designated by the manufacturer.

Q26. a) What effect does orangeflower water have when used in a facial mask? *(2 marks)*
b) When would distilled or mineral water be chosen as a liquid ingredient rather than rosewater and witch-hazel? *(2 marks)*

Answer:
a) Orangeflower water has a noticeable astringent effect, tightens pores and tones the skin.
b) Water would be chosen if the therapist wanted to achieve the effects of treatment from the dry mask ingredients only. Water is often chosen for more delicate skins or skins which can be unpredictable during treatment.

Q27. What are the benefits and effects of a non-setting mask? *(6 marks)*

Answer:
Benefits Include:
• Does not harden or tighten on the skin, so very useful for clients who are claustrophobic or do not like the tightening action of setting masks.
• Easier to remove than setting masks because they are in gel or cream form; beneficial for use on skins that are a little loose.

• Some products are 'fast acting' so treatment times can be reduced. Ideal for clients with limited time.
• Can be purchased ready prepared; this can be useful in a busy salon and could lead to a possible sale for home care use.

Effects include:
• A full range of effects can be produced, depending on the mask ingredients chosen, eg firming, pH balancing, stimulating, rejuvenating.
• Sensitive skins can be treated (using the appropriate product).
• Generally refining and desquamative.

Q28. What type of skin would benefit from a paraffin wax mask treatment?

(2 marks)

Answer:
Possible Answer 1 – any skin would benefit from a paraffin wax treatment except for:
1. Infected acne conditions.
2. Infected skin.
3. Generally florid skins or skins that are easily stimulated.
4. Skins with excessive broken capillaries.
5. Hypersensitive skins.

Possible Answer 2 – dry, mature skin or skin with a lot of facial lines would benefit from a paraffin wax treatment. Also oily skin or unbalanced skin would benefit from the stabilising desquamative effect of this treatment. This treatment can also be used as a preventative treatment on a younger, dryer skin type, or on most skin types in need of deep cleansing and stimulation, providing no heat sensitivity or broken capillaries are present.

Q29. Give an example of the use of paraffin wax treatments, other than in a facial mask. *(2 marks)*

Answer: In a deluxe manicure or pedicure treatment, to improve dry skin and nails and improve circulation to the limbs.

Q30. a) What is meant by the term 'a biological mask'? *(1 mark)*
b) Give *two* examples of a biological mask and state what type of skin they are appropriate for. *(4 marks)*

Answer:

a) A biological mask is made from natural products, eg fruit, food, plants or herbs.

b) • Dry skin mask – yolk of an egg mixed with almond oil.

• Oily skin mask – beaten egg white mixed with a few drops of lemon juice.

• Mature skin mask – one spoonful of warmed honey mixed with a few drops of lemon or orange juice.

• Oily, coarse skin mask – mashed cucumber mixed with three drops of orangeflower water and three drops of orange or lemon juice, applied over a layer of gauze.

CLIENT SCENARIOS

In this section, completed record cards detailing beauty therapy treatments are provided for you to review. You will then be asked a series of questions about the treatments that took place. An example answer is also provided.

This type of testing helps to improve your skills in treatment planning. It is also a different, yet realistic, way of testing and will definitely help you to think about how accurately you complete record cards!

Skin Care Record Card – Example One

This record card clearly details the client's current home care routine, or should I say, lack of home care routine!

This client is a smoker and a cold sore sufferer, is allergic to fish and has acne-type scarring. Being allergic to fish is a common allergy, and care should be taken with clients suffering from this allergy when using some products of marine extract.

Also some clients who are cold sore sufferers report that ozone steaming can influence a cold sore breakout. The client described in Example One would certainly have benefited from an ozone steaming treatment, but vapour steaming was chosen instead to be on the safe side.

Overall this record card was completed fully and the treatments chosen were appropriate. The pore release massage routine was a good suggestion for the client's acne-type scarring.

SKIN CARE RECORD CARD

Name: _____ DOB _____

Address: _____

_____

GP Name and Address: _____

Telephone Home: _____

Telephone Work: _____

Can be contacted   Yes ☐   No ☐

Client Ref Code: _____

Client Signature _____

Therapist Signature _____

Date: _____

Contra-Indications: Heart conditions ☐   Diabetes ☐   Epilepsy ☐   Eczema ☐   Psoriasis ☐   Recent surgery ☐

Scar tissue ☐   Known allergies: _____   Medication: _____   Other: _____

Other information: Sensitive eyes ☐   Sensitive skin ☐   Cold sore sufferer ☐   Smoker ☐   Lack of skin sensation ☐

Details of Current Skin Care:

Skin Analysis	Massage
Main Treatment Needs/Plan	Mask Therapy
Cleansing	Specialist Products
Exfoliating	Moisturising
Steaming	Aftercare/Home care
	Other Comments

SKIN CARE RECORD CARD – Example One

Name: Diane Daniels	DOB 20.10.70	Telephone Home: 12345	Client Ref Code: DD11

Address: 8 The Pines | Telephone Work: 78910 | Client Signature *D Daniels*

North Cheshire | Can be contacted Yes ☑ No ☐ | Therapist Signature *J Smith*

GP Name and Address: Dr Taylor, The Surgery, Cheshire | Date: 1.10.2002

Contra-Indications:

Heart conditions ☒   Diabetes ☒   Epilepsy ☒   Eczema ☒   Psoriasis ☒   Recent surgery ☒

Scar tissue ☑   Known allergies: Fish   Medication: None   Other:

Other information:

Sensitive eyes ☒   Sensitive skin ☒   Cold sore sufferer ☑   Smoker ☑   Lack of skin sensation ☒

Details of Current Skin Care:

Uses a wash off cleanser from local drugstore, an astringent to tone. Moisturises now and then with a moisturising cream, puts tea tree oil on spots, has an occasional mask which she buys for an oily skin type.

Skin Analysis Oily skin, coarse texture, open pores, shiny all over, generally poor appearance, complexion dull and lifeless, many breakouts and comedones in the nose, chin and cheek areas. Evidence of fine lines appearing around the mouth. A few acne scars present.

Massage Light pore release routine duration 16 minutes; skin quite pink following treatment. Corrective treatment oil from Oily Balance Range – No 2 formula. General relaxing effleurage and petrissage on the shoulders.

Main Treatment Needs/Plan Client requests help in eliminating comedones, would like to improve the appearance of the skin and reduce breakouts, also control the oiliness. Aim to deep cleanse, extractions, pore cleansing massage and mask, provide advice on better home care regime.

Mask Therapy Mask of one part kaolin, one part magnesium, one part calamine mixed with rosewater, duration six minutes.

Cleansing Eye make-up remover. Double cleanse – once with cleansing emulsion, once with cleansing wash and soft pore brush. Toning with witch hazel.

Specialist Products Oil-absorbing moisturiser from Oily Balance Range – slightly tinted formula.

Exfoliating None today.

Moisturising Oily balance tinted (control).

Steaming Vapour steaming only. 50 cms distance. Eye pads applied. Time to produce slight erythema. Nine minutes (skin colour good). Extractions around nose and chin. (Not very successful, comedones well established.)

Aftercare/Home care Advice documented on consultation sheet. Advised to use cleanser, toner & light moisturiser daily from Oily Balance range or similar. Advised wash off cleanser not sufficient. Sampled with 'oil absorbing moisturiser tinted'.

Other Comments Advised to stop using neat tea tree oil on spots, and exfoliate every week. Discussed the long term benefits of regular facials and explained comedones may take a few visits to remove completely. Client booked for the following week.

EXAMPLE ONE, SHORT ANSWER QUESTIONS

Q1. How does a 'pore release' massage routine differ from a general routine?

Answer: A pore release routine is not a relaxing sedative routine, but is designed to free the pores of sebaceous secretions, and thoroughly deep cleanse the skin. The effect of the treatment is to refine surface texture and produce erythema. There is no real effect on the facial muscles, but acne scarring can be improved and oily secretions can be more easily controlled with regular treatments. The routine involves a lot of compression movements linked up by gentle effleurage and lymph drainage movements.

Q2. Explain why specialist active treatment products were not chosen for this client.

Answer: The client had an unsophisticated skin care routine. The use of specialist active products could have caused a reaction as they might have been too intensive for the skin. These products could be introduced on subsequent visits with confidence.

Q3. a) What would be the action of the mask ingredient kaolin chosen for this client as part of her treatment mask?
b) Why was kaolin chosen as a mask ingredient above fuller's earth, which is renowned for its deep cleansing, drawing and stimulating effect?

Answer:
a) Kaolin has a deep cleansing and stimulating action on the skin.
b) The client received a stimulating pore release massage treatment. The skin was quite pink following treatment. Fuller's earth would have been too stimulating a mask ingredient for use at this time.

Q4. Outline three benefits of using a wash-off cleanser and soft pore brush on this client.

Answer: The wash-off cleanser could have been chosen because the client was familiar with this type of product. The wash-off cleanser used with a pore brush would have been gently exfoliating for the skin. The pore brush would have loosened dead skin cells in areas of comedones which were to be extracted later in the treatment.

Q5. As part of the home care advice, the client was advised to exfoliate weekly. What are the advantages of using such a product at home?

Answer: Exfoliating products remove dead skin cells so the skin appears more glowing following their use. Using such a product at home would enhance the effect of cosmetic products applied to the skin because they would be able to work more effectively. Also, keeping the skin's surface free of dead layers and debris allows the skin to function more effectively.

Q6. State two possible causes of overactive sebaceous glands.

Answer:
• Hormonal control – too many hormones circulating in the blood stream, eg puberty.
• Drugs/medication – certain drugs can cause this problem, eg contraceptive pills, drugs that affect metabolism.

Q7. How does smoking affect the skin?

Answer: Smoking has a negative effect on the skin. The nicotine in cigarettes causes constriction of the blood vessels which can increase blood pressure and lead to heart conditions. This constriction of blood vessels has the effect of reducing nutrient supply to the skin which can cause the skin to age prematurely, suffer broken capillaries and spider veins, and even display an unsightly mottled appearance.

Carbon monoxide is also found within inhaled cigarette smoke. Blood cells have a higher affinity or attraction to carbon monoxide than oxygen. This means that in smokers less oxygen is transported to the cells, which also affects cell nutrition and cell renewal and the outward appearance of the skin.

Inhaled cigarette smoke contains free radicals. Free radicals are simply loose ions or particles that can irritate the lumen of blood vessels affecting circulation even further. Free radicals also cause other unpleasant diseases.

SKIN CARE RECORD CARD – Example Two

Name: Ellen Robertson **DOB** 6.4.1940 **Telephone Home:** 891011 **Client Ref Code:** ER 1

Address: Jonquil House, Cumbria

Telephone Work: Retired **Client Signature** *Ellen Robertson*

Can be contacted Yes ☑ No ☐ **Therapist Signature** *M Whyte*

GP Name and Address: Dr Young, The Surgery, Cumbria **Date:** 24.7.2001

Contra-Indications:
Heart conditions ☒ **Diabetes** ☒ **Epilepsy** ☒ **Eczema** ☒ **Psoriasis** ☒ **Recent surgery** ☒

Scar tissue ☒ **Known allergies:** Strawberries **Medication:** None **Other:** Client allergic to many cosmetics in the past. Has not had allergy testing.

Other information:
Sensitive eyes ☑ **Sensitive skin** ☑ *Soap **Cold sore sufferer** ☑ **Smoker** ☑ **Lack of skin sensation** ☒

Details of Current Skin Care:
Very good skin care regime, regular facials, quality products. Uses cleansers, toners, specialist firming products, treatment creams. Can be sensitive to soap, and highly-perfumed products cause reactions. Not sensitive to heat.

Skin Analysis Dry skin, signs of maturity, jowls, gentle sagging appearance, lines established around neck, eyes, corrugator and forehead. Fine, even texture, colour good, skin extremely soft. No age spots, tags etc. No comedones or milium, no broken capillaries.

Massage Brief ten minutes massage on the decollette (a lot of emphasis on the upper arms), only superficial effleurage on the face, gentle eye-lifting circles. Massage medium 'super rich massage cream'.

Main Treatment Needs/Plan Client booked for a paraffin wax mask treatment. Aim to soften lines, moisturise, refine.

Mask Therapy Paraffin wax mask over layer of 'massage medium' left until cool – 14 minutes duration. Skin slightly pink following treatment, glowing, lines a little softer.

Cleansing Eye and lip make-up remover. Double cleanse using treatment cleansing cream with ginseng. Toning with rosewater on dampened c/w.

Specialist Products Hypoallergenic eye cream applied to the eyes during treatment. Firming ampule applied under the massage medium.

Exfoliating None today.

Moisturising Light application of tinted moisturiser – colour soft beige.

Steaming None today.

Aftercare/Home care No make-up for 12 hours to be applied. Continue with current home care regime.

Other Comments Client satisfied with the result. Recommended to have a paraffin wax mask monthly. Client advised to include paraffin wax treatments in her hand care programme.

Skin Care Record Card – Example Two

This record card was for a more mature client who was having a restricted facial, ie, not too many treatments could be performed prior to the paraffin wax mask, thus avoiding over stimulation of the skin.

You will note that the client described had an excellent skin care routine, was a little sensitive and allergic, but not heat sensitive. She reacted to highly-perfumed products, which is quite common.

The client had no high colouring or broken veins, and wanted to soften facial lines. The paraffin wax mask was a suitable choice for her. A hot oil mask would also have been another alternative.

Applying the moisturising massage treatment cream under the mask would have further enhanced the treatment, so again was a good choice of product.

EXAMPLE TWO, SHORT ANSWER QUESTIONS

Q1. The client was described as having 'jowls'. What facial muscles contribute to the appearance of jowls?

Answer:
- The platysma.
- The depressors of the lower lip, especially the triangularis muscle.
- The masseter.

Q2. Which muscle causes horizontal lines to appear across the top of the nose when tone is lost?

Answer: The procerus.

Q3. Which muscle causes a 'drooping eyes' appearance when tone is lost?

Answer: The orbicularis oculi.

Q4. What type of mask treatment should this client avoid?

Answer: A biological mask treatment that involves the use of soft fruit, especially strawberries.

Q5. List four effects of a paraffin wax mask.

Answer:
- Skin perspiration is greatly enhanced.
- Surface adhesions are released.
- Gentle desquamation occurs.
- Products applied under the mask are more readily absorbed.
- Superficial circulation is increased.
- The deeper epidermis layers are regenerated.
- Lines and wrinkles appear softer.
- Skin texture and appearance appears fresher.

Q6. What muscle covers the shoulder joint and would have been included in the massage of the decollette?

Answer: The deltoid.

Q7. Name the other muscles of the shoulder girdle that would have been included in this facial massage, and state where they are positioned.

Answer:
- The trapezius, a large flat triangular muscle covering the upper back and sides and back of the neck.
- The pectorals, two fan-shaped muscles found in the upper chest region on the front of the body, from the middle of the body to the upper arm.

Q8. What are milium?

Answer: Milia or milium are commonly called whiteheads. Whiteheads occur when sebum is trapped in a blind follicle. It cannot escape, so forms a hard pearly lump just below the skin's surface.

Skin Care Record Card – Example Three

By now you should be able to see where record cards have not been completed as fully as they should be.

Example Three is quite detailed. This client enjoyed an appropriate facial, but the aftercare was a little weak. It states that advice was given about specialist products and their use, but it does not tell us what specialist products were discussed. The record card tells us what ranges were used, eg mature range or sensi range. This was a plus point. Also this client had no contra-indications or

SKIN CARE RECORD CARD – Example Three

Name: Lynda Mellers   DOB 24.7.47   **Telephone Home:** 12345   **Client Ref Code:** LM 9

Address: The Grange   **Telephone Work:** 78910   **Client Signature** *Lynda Mellers*

West Midlands B21   **Can be contacted** Yes ☑ No ☐   **Therapist Signature** *D Cheedle*

GP Name and Address: Dr Brown. The Surgery, B21   **Date:** 1.5.2001

Contra-Indications:

Heart conditions ☒   Diabetes ☒   Epilepsy ☒   Eczema ☑   Psoriasis ☒   Recent surgery ☒

Scar tissue ☒   **Known allergies:** None   **Medication:** None   **Other:** Sometimes gets a little eczema on the feet if stressed.

Other information:

Sensitive eyes ☑   Sensitive skin ☒   Cold sore sufferer ☒   Smoker ☒   Lack of skin sensation ☒

Details of Current Skin Care:

Has a regular routine, uses quality products, always uses hypoallergenic eye make-up remover, exfoliates monthly, uses a mask monthly, no special night products used or anti-ageing products.

Skin Analysis Good appearance, small pores, even texture, has lines around the eyes and neck, overall slightly dry, facial contours slightly relaxed around naso-labial area. Skin colour good. Skin around eyes a little dry. | **Massage** Emphasis neck, eyes and middle face, extra lifting and circles. Duration full 20 minutes. Massage medium – treatment cream from Mature range.

Main Treatment Needs/Plan (Client wants an anti-ageing facial.) Light exfoliation, emphasis on massage to lift naso-labial folds, soften lines in neck and eye area. Correct dryness of the eyes using suitable product and light massage to soften lines. Mask using clay ingredients but non-setting. Give home care advice about anti-ageing products. | **Mask Therapy** Calamine, magnesium and almond oil – 10 minutes duration. Cooling eye pads applied during the mask dampened with witch-hazel.

Cleansing Eye make-up remover gel from Sensi range. Double cleanse using cream dermafloral toner from the Mature range. | **Specialist Products** De-sensitising serum patted around eye contour. Firming serum applied under the massage cream. Lifting and toning serum applied under moisturiser.

Exfoliating Exfoliating cream (Mature range) left on skin four minutes. Remove warm sponges. | **Moisturising** Eye cream around eyes (Sensi range). Light moisturiser from Mature range.

Steaming None today. | **Aftercare/Home care** Advice given about specialist treatment products and their use. Sample given of night cream from Mature range.

Other Comments Recommended and discussed having a paraffin wax treatment at another visit. Client commented she found the witch-hazel eye pads a little irritating. Review this next time.

special requirements that might have made the treatment a little more difficult to plan.

EXAMPLE THREE, SHORT ANSWER QUESTIONS

Q1. The skin analysis revealed a dry skin with relaxed contours around the naso-labial fold. In a dry skin which glands are under-producing?

Answer: The sebaceous glands.

Q2. Where are these glands situated?

Answer: In the dermis.

Q3. Which muscles contribute to the condition known as 'naso-labial folds'?

Answer: The levator quadratus muscles.

Q4. During cleansing a dermafloral toning lotion was used. What advantages would the use of this product have, if any?

Answer: This type of toning product would be alcohol free, and would derive its toning and degreasing action on the skin by the use of its plant or herbal ingredients. It would be appropriate for this skin type because the skin is dry, and it would not dry the skin further.

Q5. What were the advantages of using specialist serums as part of this facial treatment?

Answer: The serums detailed on the record card are aimed to treat specific needs of the client. The desensitising serum would desensitise the eye contour area, whilst other serums were chosen to lift and firm the skin. The client requested an anti-ageing facial. These products would contribute to meeting the needs of the client and the overall treatment plan.

Q6. A mask of calamine magnesium and almond oil was used on the client.
a) What is the action of the mask ingredient magnesium?
b) What type of oil is almond oil?
c) What liquid mask ingredient would be suitable for this client if she requested a setting mask?

Answer:

a) Magnesium has a mild toning action and is slightly desquamative.

b) Almond oil is derived from almonds so is really a nut oil. It is sometimes classed as a vegetable oil.

c) Rosewater, water, or a mixture of both.

Q7. The client commented she found the witch-hazel eye pads a little irritating. Give a suitable alternative.

Answer: The eyes are sensitive and dry, so a suitable alternative would be to apply a cooling hypoallergenic eye gel under the eye pads dampened with water, or a diluted mild dermafloral lotion.

FINAL END TEST

This section consists of statements. Each one may be correct or incorrect. The answer required is simply

Yes or No

In your assessment of whether the statement is correct or incorrect, you must only base your answer on the information provided. The answers can be located on pages 218–220.

• FINAL END TEST

1. The mandible is the only moveable bone of the skull.

2. The upper jaw bones are called the maxillae.

3. Another name for the cheek bone is the zygomatic bone.

4. The temporal bone is pierced by the foramen magnus.

5. There are three parietal bones.

6. The occipital bone is situated at the back of the head.

⬭

7. The frontal, zygomatic and nasal bones contribute to an individual's face shape.

⬭

8. The platysma is a facial muscle.

⬭

9. The sterno mastoid muscles nod the head.

⬭

10. The procerus is a sphincter muscle.

⬭

11. The masseter is an important muscle for the mastication process.

⬭

12. The buccinator is found in the cheek area.

⬭

13. The obicularis oris surrounds the eye.

⬭

14. When the platysma loses tone, it causes a wrinkled neck.

⬭

15. There are *three* levators of the upper lip.

⬭

16. The scapulae are found at the back of the body.

⬭

17. The clavicles are sometimes called the collar bones.

⬭

18. Another name for the breast bone is the sternum.

⬭

19. The deltoid muscle helps to rotate the arm.

⬭

20. The pectorals are found at the back of the body.

⬭

21. The trapezius is a large triangular muscle.

⬭

22. The deltoid helps rotate the arm.

⬭

23. The trapezius helps to rotate the arm.

⬭

24. Talcum powder comes under COSHH regulations.

25. Oils like almond and grapeseed can go off and become rancid.

26. Massage cream is a popular medium for oily skins.

27. Active massage products like serums and ampules can be applied under the massage cream/oil.

28. Percussion movements are really tapotement movements.

29. Tapotement movements should be used liberally on thin clients.

30. Compression movements relax larger muscles.

31. Effleurage movements are stroking movements.

32. Massage is performed in a centripetal direction for best effect.

33. Vibration is useful on clients with a loose skin.

34. Conjuctivitis is a contra-indication to facial treatments.

35. Skin tags and warts can be avoided during massage treatments.

36. Vascular areas would contra-indicate any facial treatments.

37. Clients who are unwell or on antibiotics normally improve following a relaxing facial.

38. Regular massage improves skin tone and colour.

39. Massage aids desquamation.

40. Elimination and absorption are enhanced by massage.

41. Calamine powder is sometimes called china clay.

42. Kaolin has a stimulating and cleansing effect on the skin.

43. Magnesium is light and toning in action.

44. The colour of fuller's earth is white.

45. Fuller's earth is useful for refining oily, coarse skin.

46. Sulphur must be used with care as it is very strong in action.

47. Witch-hazel is normally used with the milder mask ingredients.

48. Rosewater is used in mask ingredients for its mild toning action.

49. Non-setting masks can come in cream or gel form and do not harden on the skin.

50. Biological masks can be made from natural fruits.

51. Biological masks have different effects depending on what fruit or products are used.

52. Thermal masks can be used on couperose skins.

53. Thermal masks are very effective on dry, lined skin conditions.

54. Peel-off masks peel off the dead skin cells when they are removed.

55. Paraffin wax masks are really biological masks.

56. Paraffin wax masks have the effect of being desquamative and softening to the skin's surface.

57. A crepey lined skin would benefit from a paraffin wax mask.

58. A hot oil mask is suitable for dry skin conditions and to improve facial colour and texture.

59. The heat source for hot oil mask treatments must be serviced regularly.

60. During a hot oil mask treatment, the client can be left unattended.

61. Lymph from the left side of the head and neck empties into the left subclavian vein.

62. The main vein which drains blood from the face and neck is called the jugular vein.

63. Arteries carry oxygenated blood to the tissues.

64. Veins are thicker than arteries and contain a series of valves. They subdivide into arterioles.

65. The facial artery supplies the upper and lower lips.

FINAL END TEST **ANSWERS**

1. Yes
2. Yes
3. Yes
4. No   The occipital bone is pierced by the foramen magnus.
5. No   There are only two – they form the dome of the skull.
6. Yes
7. Yes
8. No   The platysma is found in the neck region.
9. Yes
10. No   The Procerus is a thin muscle found between the eyebrows.
11. Yes
12. Yes
13. No   It surrounds the mouth.
14. Yes
15. No   There are four levators, two on each side of the face.
16. Yes
17. Yes
18. Yes
19. Yes
20. No   They are found at the front of the body and support the breasts.
21. Yes
22. Yes   Movement occurs because muscles work in harmony together.
23. Yes   Both the trapezius and deltoid help to rotate the arm.
24. Yes
25. Yes   Quite true, and the smell is very unpleasant.
26. No   Lighter textured oils are more popular, creams are more popular with dry skins.
27. Yes   This is an acceptable time to apply such products.
28. Yes
29. No   It should be restricted on thin clients as it could be painful.
30. Yes
31. Yes
32. Yes

33. Yes
34. Yes
35. Yes
36. No   Vascular areas can be omitted from treatment, and can even be improved by the use of the correct products.
37. No   If a client is unwell or taking medication, a massage can make them more unwell.
38. Yes
39. Yes
40. Yes
41. No   Kaolin is sometimes called china clay.
42. Yes
43. Yes
44. No   It is greeny-grey in colour.
45. Yes
46. Yes
47. No   It is normally used with the stronger mask ingredients, because it is quite astringent.
48. Yes
49. Yes
50. Yes
51. Yes
52. No   They would worsen a couperose skin.
53. Yes
54. Yes
55. No   Quite untrue. Paraffin wax is made from ingredients like mineral oil, paraffin wax and beeswax, not from fruits or plants. Also paraffin wax does harden or set on the skin; biological masks do not.
56. Yes
57. Yes
58. Yes
59. Yes
60. No   This must *never* happen in case of accident. It would be in breach of the Health and Safety at Work Act.

61. Yes
62. Yes
63. Yes
64. No   Veins are thinner than arteries but they do contain valves. They subdivide into venules not arteries.

65. Yes

Marking Guide and Grading

Check your answers and then check them against the guide below. In percentage terms, 60% is considered a pass. With this type of end test, because it's a simple Yes or No answer, there is a strong likelihood you could have guessed some of the answers! You should take this into account when determining your grade.

Above 59 correct   answers is exceptional!

52 correct   credit – excellent

39 correct   pass – well done

Below 39 correct answers means you need to spend more time revising, so go back to your course notes and Revision Maps, and then have another go.

CHAPTER FIVE

LASH AND BROW TREATMENTS

CHECKLIST ✓ Can You?

	Yes	No	Page No
1. State the contra-indications to eyebrow shaping.			222
2. Provide guidelines for choosing eyebrow shapes.			223
3. Discuss hygiene and client care requirements for eyebrow shaping.			224
4. State the contra-indications to lash and brow tinting.			225
5. Give the safety precautions for lash and brow tinting.			226
6. State the contra-indications and safety precautions for the application of false eyelashes.			227
7. Write about the products used in the treatments covered in this chapter.			229
8. Attempt a final end test.			239

LASH AND BROW TREATMENTS

Eye treatments are a small but very important beauty therapy service. It is much more realistic to test this area practically, but questions do occasionally appear on test papers and in examinations. Naturally, theory questions tend to focus around the recognition factors of contra-indications, hygiene, sterilisation and patch testing.

Short answer questions are provided on page 230. Some multiple-choice questions are included to enable you to practice and check your progress; finally an end test will assist your revision and provide additional examination practice.

Revision Map – Contra-indications to Eyebrow Shaping

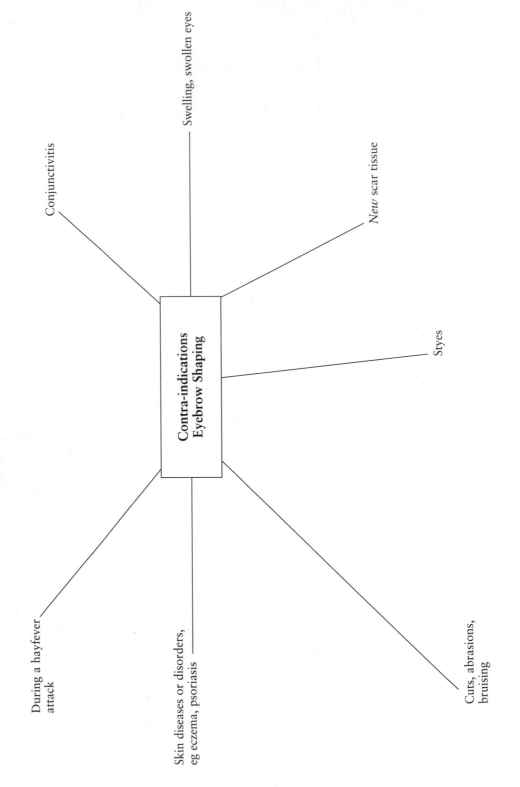

Conjunctivitis

Swelling, swollen eyes

During a hayfever attack

**Contra-indications
Eyebrow Shaping**

Skin diseases or disorders, eg eczema, psoriasis

New scar tissue

Styes

Cuts, abrasions, bruising

Revision Map – Choosing Eyebrow Shapes

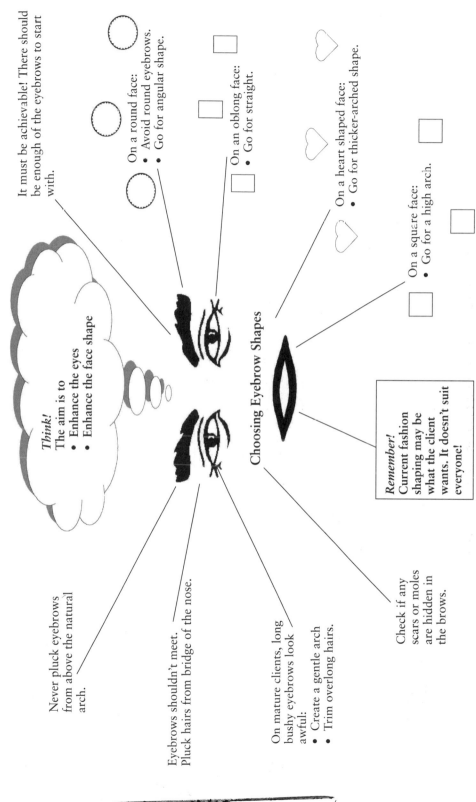

Think!
The aim is to
- Enhance the eyes
- Enhance the face shape

It must be achievable! There should be enough of the eyebrows to start with.

On a round face:
- Avoid round eyebrows.
- Go for angular shape.

On an oblong face:
- Go for straight.

On a heart shaped face:
- Go for thicker-arched shape.

On a square face:
- Go for a high arch.

Choosing Eyebrow Shapes

Remember!
Current fashion shaping may be what the client wants. It doesn't suit everyone!

Check if any scars or moles are hidden in the brows.

On mature clients, long bushy eyebrows look awful:
- Create a gentle arch
- Trim overlong hairs.

Eyebrows shouldn't meet. Pluck hairs from bridge of the nose.

Never pluck eyebrows from above the natural arch.

Revision Map – Hygiene and Client Care for Eyebrow Shaping Treatments

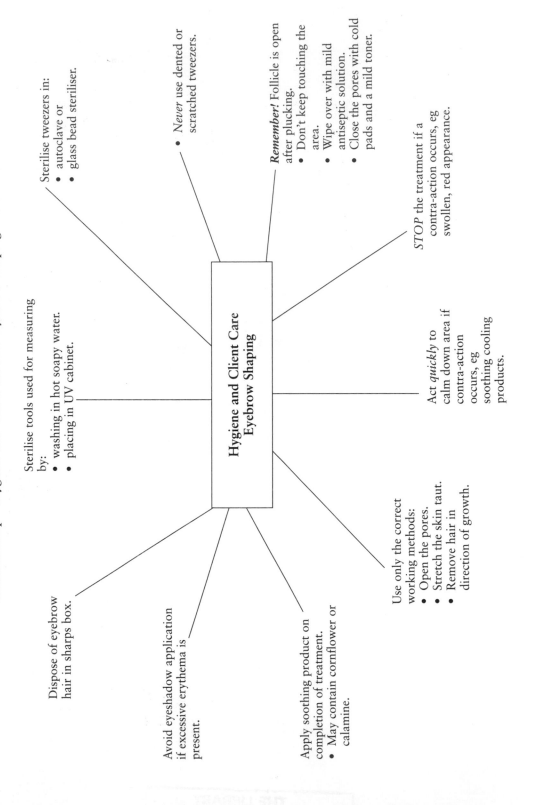

Sterilise tweezers in:
- autoclave or
- glass bead steriliser.

- *Never* use dented or scratched tweezers.

Remember! Follicle is open after plucking.
- Don't keep touching the area.
- Wipe over with mild antiseptic solution.
- Close the pores with cold pads and a mild toner.

STOP the treatment if a contra-action occurs, eg swollen, red appearance.

Sterilise tools used for measuring by:
- washing in hot soapy water.
- placing in UV cabinet.

Hygiene and Client Care Eyebrow Shaping

Act *quickly* to calm down area if contra-action occurs, eg soothing cooling products.

Dispose of eyebrow hair in sharps box.

Avoid eyeshadow application if excessive erythema is present.

Apply soothing product on completion of treatment.
- May contain cornflower or calamine.

Use only the correct working methods:
- Open the pores.
- Stretch the skin taut.
- Remove hair in direction of growth.

Revision Map – Contra-indications to Lash and Brow Tinting

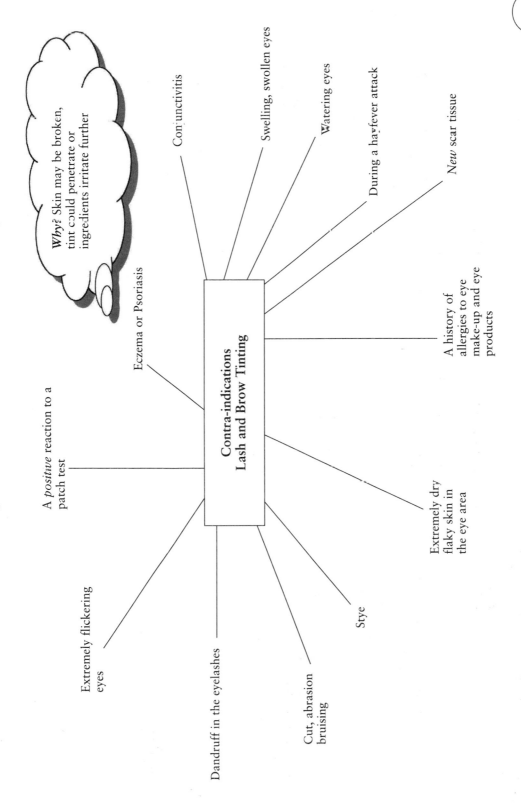

Why? Skin may be broken, tint could penetrate or ingredients irritate further

Conjunctivitis

Swelling, swollen eyes

Watering eyes

During a hayfever attack

New scar tissue

A history of allergies to eye make-up and eye products

Eczema or Psoriasis

**Contra-indications
Lash and Brow Tinting**

A *positive* reaction to a patch test

Extremely dry flaky skin in the eye area

Extremely flickering eyes

Stye

Dandruff in the eyelashes

Cut, abrasion bruising

Revision Map – Safety Precautions for Lash and Brow Tinting

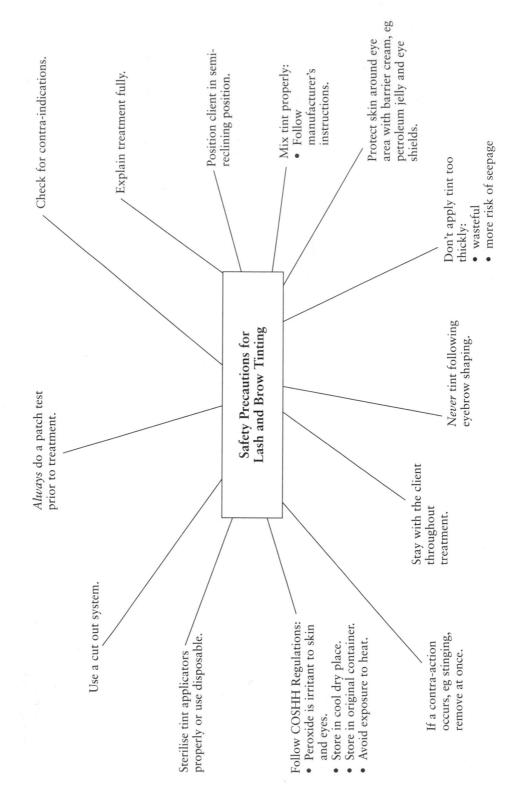

Check for contra-indications.

Explain treatment fully.

Position client in semi-reclining position.

Mix tint properly:
- Follow manufacturer's instructions.

Protect skin around eye area with barrier cream, eg petroleum jelly and eye shields.

Don't apply tint too thickly:
- wasteful
- more risk of seepage

Always do a patch test prior to treatment.

Safety Precautions for Lash and Brow Tinting

Never tint following eyebrow shaping.

Use a cut out system.

Sterilise tint applicators properly or use disposable.

Follow COSHH Regulations:
- Peroxide is irritant to skin and eyes.
- Store in cool dry place.
- Store in original container.
- Avoid exposure to heat.

If a contra-action occurs, eg stinging, remove at once.

Stay with the client throughout treatment.

Revision Map – Contra-indications to the Application of False Eyelashes

Any eye infections
- Conjunctivitis.
- Stye.

Watery eye conditions

During hayfever attack

Extremely dry flaky skin in eye area

Hypersensitivity in the eye area

Contra-indications to False Eyelashes

Swelling, cut, abrasion

A *positive* reaction to the patch test

Eczema
Psoriasis

Previous allergic reaction to eyelash adhesive or solvent

Revision Map – Safety Precautions for the Application of False Eye Lashes

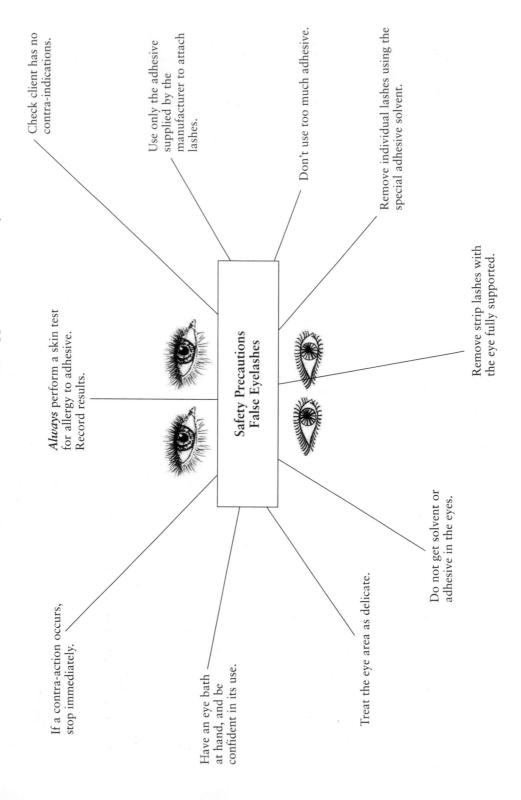

Check client has no contra-indications.

Use only the adhesive supplied by the manufacturer to attach lashes.

Don't use too much adhesive.

Remove individual lashes using the special adhesive solvent.

Remove strip lashes with the eye fully supported.

Always perform a skin test for allergy to adhesive. Record results.

Safety Precautions False Eyelashes

If a contra-action occurs, stop immediately.

Have an eye bath at hand, and be confident in its use.

Treat the eye area as delicate.

Do not get solvent or adhesive in the eyes.

Revision Map – Products in Use, Eyebrow Shaping Lash and Brow Tinting and False Lash Application

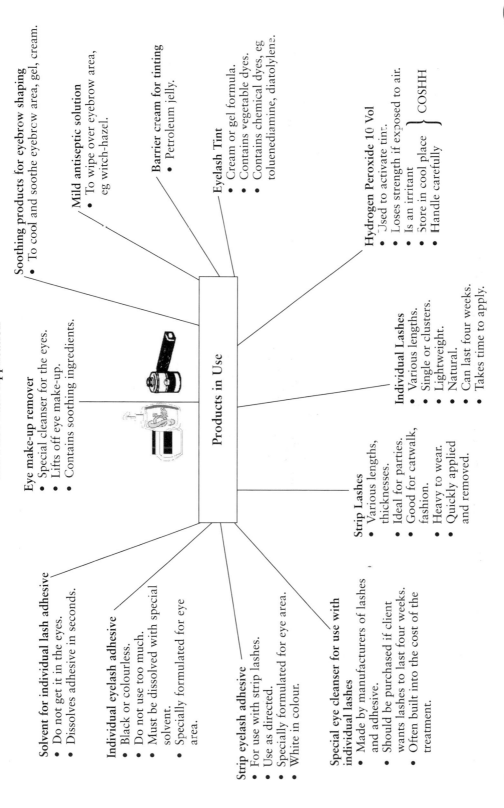

Products in Use

Soothing products for eyebrow shaping
- To cool and soothe eyebrow area, gel, cream.

Mild antiseptic solution
- To wipe over eyebrow area, eg witch-hazel.

Barrier cream for tinting
- Petroleum jelly.

Eyelash Tint
- Cream or gel formula.
- Contains vegetable dyes.
- Contains chemical dyes, eg toluenediamine, diatolylene.

Hydrogen Peroxide 10 Vol
- Used to activate tint.
- Loses strength if exposed to air. ⎫
- Is an irritant   ⎬ COSHH
- Store in cool place   ⎭
- Handle carefully

Eye make-up remover
- Special cleanser for the eyes.
- Lifts off eye make-up.
- Contains soothing ingredients.

Individual Lashes
- Various lengths.
- Single or clusters.
- Lightweight.
- Natural.
- Can last four weeks.
- Takes time to apply.

Strip Lashes
- Various lengths, thicknesses.
- Ideal for parties.
- Good for catwalk, fashion.
- Heavy to wear.
- Quickly applied and removed.

Solvent for individual lash adhesive
- Do not get it in the eyes.
- Dissolves adhesive in seconds.

Individual eyelash adhesive
- Black or colourless.
- Do not use too much.
- Must be dissolved with special solvent.
- Specially formulated for eye area.

Strip eyelash adhesive
- For use with strip lashes.
- Use as directed.
- Specially formulated for eye area.
- White in colour.

Special eye cleanser for use with individual lashes
- Made by manufacturers of lashes and adhesive.
- Should be purchased if client wants lashes to last four weeks.
- Often built into the cost of the treatment.

1 Eyebrow shaping

Revision Maps focused around choosing eyebrow shapes, hygiene and client care are provided to help prompt your revision (see pages 222–224).

2. Lash and Brow Tinting

See pages 225–226 for Revision Maps focused around contra-indications and safety precautions.

You should also look carefully at the Revision Map on page 229, focusing on products used to carry out eye treatments; there are important references to eyelash tinting products that should be included in your revision.

3. False Eyelashes and products in use

Revision Maps focused around contra-indications, safety precautions and products used in eye treatments are provided on pages 227–228 to prompt your revision.

SHORT ANSWER QUESTIONS

An example of some model questions and answers are provided to help give you an insight on how to answer questions properly. Reading through the questions and answers will also help your revision.

Q1. What action should be taken if a contra-action occurred during eyebrow shaping and the eyebrow became very red and swollen? *(4 marks)*

Answer: The treatment must be stopped at once, and cold compresses should be applied to the area. The client should be kept calm by the therapist and reassured that the reaction will subside. A soothing antiseptic product should be applied to the area. The client should be advised to apply a soothing product at intervals for the next 48 hours.

Q2. What is the *best* way to sterilise tweezers? *(1 mark)*

Answer: In an autoclave.

Q3. How should tweezers be sterilised if an autoclave or glass bead steriliser was not available? *(2 marks)*

Answer: The tweezers could be wiped over with surgical spirit and placed in a UV cabinet. They should be exposed to the UV rays for 15 minutes each side.

Q4. Why is *immersion* a less popular method of sterilising tweezers? *(1 mark)*

Answer: Regular immersion could lead to rusting of the tweezers.

Q5. If a client had strong eyebrow hair and wanted a reshaping treatment, how can the therapist minimise client discomfort? *(4 marks)*

Answer:
• By warming the area beforehand using hot compresses or even a facial steamer.
• By holding the skin taut during treatment and plucking in the direction of the hair growth.
• By regularly wiping over the area with warm compresses during treatment.
• By using automatic tweezers if available.
• By putting the client at ease before and during treatment.

Q6. Outline the appearance of conjunctivitis. *(1 mark)*

Answer: The eyes appear very red and irritated. They are watery and often ooze pus.

Q7. Define the eye condition conjunctivitis. *(2 marks)*

Answer: This is a bacterial infection that inflames the mucous membrane of the eye and lining of the eyelids. It is infectious and extremely unpleasant for the sufferer.

Q8. Under COSHH regulations how should hydrogen peroxide be stored? *(2 marks)*

Answer: In a cool cupboard in its original container.

Q9. Why does hydrogen peroxide fall under COSHH regulations? *(1 mark)*

Answer: Because it is an irritant product.

Q10. Why must eyebrow shaping *always* follow any tinting treatment? *(2 marks)*

Answer: Tinting of the lashes or brows is always carried out first, because when eyebrow hair is plucked from the follicle, the follicle remains slightly open and disturbed. Any tint or peroxide entering the follicle could quite easily result in an unpleasant reaction or irritation for the client.

Q11. Why must a test patch be carried out 24–48 hours before treatment?

(2 marks)

Answer: A skin test or patch test is carried out to determine if the client is suitable for treatment. An adverse reaction to the skin test would mean the treatment should not go ahead. The skin's chemistry can change very quickly, so the test should be carried out 24–48 hours before the treatment is scheduled.

Q12. Does a *negative* response to the skin test *guarantee* the client could not suffer a reaction? Justify your answer. *(5 marks)*

Answer: No, but it shows that the therapist has 'taken due care' which is very important should the client attempt to bring a legal case against the salon. A reaction is less likely to occur if no reaction to the skin test took place. However, the chemistry of the skin changes rapidly and the test is carried out on skin behind the ear or the elbow, not the skin of the delicate eye area. It would be inadvisable for the therapist to guarantee totally that no reaction could occur.

Q13. What would be a suitable colour for a natural redhead requesting an eyelash and brow tint? The client is very apprehensive about the treatment and wants a natural look. Justify your answer. *(2 marks)*

Answer: Brown would be a safe colour to recommend to the client. The effect would look natural but would darken the lash and brow hairs to give definition to the eyes.

Q14. Which type of dyes are found in lash tinting products? *(2 marks)*

Answer: Vegetable dye and safe chemical dye (eg diatolulene) are commonly found in lash tinting products.

Q15. If the client has a *positive* reaction to a skin test, how does the area appear? *(2 marks)*

Answer: The area will be red, even swollen, and irritation will be present.

Q16. Why does red hair take *longer* to process in lash and brow tinting treatments? *(1 mark)*

Answer: Because red hair is extremely resistant to the tint.

Q17. What could happen if eyebrow tint containing 20 vol peroxide was applied to the client? *(2 marks)*

Answer: A serious skin reaction could occur. Hydrogen peroxide is an irritant and only 10 vol must be used for this treatment.

Q18. State four factors that could contribute to a poor lash tinting result. *(4 marks)*

Answer:
- If the peroxide had 'gone off' or lost its strength.
- There was a greasy residue or petroleum jelly on the lashes.
- The tint and peroxide was not properly mixed.
- The tint did not have enough time to process properly.

Q19. Why must eyelash tinting be carried out with the client in a semi-reclining position? *(2 marks)*

Answer: This is a health and safety requirement. If the client was lying completely flat, the tint could easily seep into the eyes.

Q20. State six contra-indications to the application of false eyelashes. *(6 marks)*

Answer:
- Hypersensitive eyes.
- Any eye infections eg conjunctivitis, styes.
- Any inflammation or swellings.
- Eczema or psoriasis in the area.
- Extremely dry flaking skin.
- If the client is allergic to the adhesive to be used.

Q21. When might strip false eyelashes be recommended to a client in preference to individual false lashes? *(5 marks)*

Answer: Strip false lashes are considered temporary and would be recommended if the client wanted to wear them for a single occasion. Strip lashes are quickly applied, need no maintenance and can be easily removed by the client at home. Individual false lashes can last up to four weeks if properly cared for. They take longer to apply and are more suitable for longer use than a single event.

Q22. How should individual false lashes be cared for at home by the client?

(2 marks)

Answer:
- The client must avoid rubbing the eye area.
- Only the specially manufactured eye make-up remover must be used to cleanse the eye area.
- Care must be taken when applying eye cosmetics, and in general a minimum amount of mascara should be used.
- The client should return to the salon to remove or add lashes.

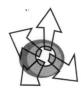

MULTIPLE CHOICE QUESTIONS

Some examples of multiple choice examination questions are included for you to enable you to give yourself a short test. Carefully consider the descriptions provided before choosing your answer. Only one answer is correct. Indicate your answer by putting an **X** in the circle: ◯

EXAMPLE
Which of the following conditions would contra-indicate an eyebrow reshape?

a) A history of allergic reaction to mascara ◯

b) A cold sore on the lower lip ◯

c) A two year old scar in the eyebrow hair ◯

d) Conjunctivitis ⊗

Correct answer is **d)**

Q1. Automatic tweezers are more appropriate when:

a) clearing a lot of eyebrow hair ◯

b) normal tweezers are not available ◯

c) tweezing hair from moles ◯

d) treating clients with a *high* pain threshold. ◯

Q2. Tweezers should *ideally* be sterilised by:

a) dipping in antiseptic solution ○

b) immersion in boiling water ○

c) an autoclave ○

d) wiping them over with witch-hazel ○

Q3. For an elderly client with bushy eyebrows, a suitable recommendation would be:

a) trim the eyebrows with scissors to ¼ inch or 6 mm length ○

b) trim overlong eyebrows and shape them into a gentle arch ○

c) shape the eyebrows to a very thin line ○

d) advise the client to remove them by waxing, and draw on a gentle arch ○

Q4. Which *hygiene* precautions should be taken on completion of an eyebrow shape?

a) wipe over the area with a mild antiseptic solution ○

b) wipe over the area with cold pads ○

c) apply cooling eye gel ○

d) wipe over the area with surgical spirit ○

Q5. On a client with a round face shape, what eyebrow shape should be avoided?

a) angular ○

b) gentle arch ○

c) rounded arch ○

d) natural arch ○

Q6. A contra-indication to eyebrow shaping is?

a) eczema in the eyebrow area ○

b) a skin tag in the area ○

c) a recent eyelash tint ○

d) migraine sufferers ○

Q7. When combining tinting and shaping treatments, the *safest* order is to:

a) tint eyebrows and lashes, book an appointment the next day for shaping ○

b) shape eyebrows, tint lashes and brows ○

c) tint then shape eyebrows, complete treatment by tinting lashes ○

d) tint eyebrows and lashes, then shape eyebrows ○

Q8. During eyebrow shaping client discomfort can be minimised by:

a) working quickly without stopping ○

b) stretching the skin taut and plucking in the direction of the hair growth ○

c) occasionally wiping over the area with a cold compress ○

d) asking the client if they are all right ○

Q9. A *positive* reaction to a tinting patch test means the client:

a) is suitable for treatment ○

b) is unsuitable for treatment ○

c) is not contra-indicated ○

d) needs a repeat patch test ○

Q10. A *positive* reaction to a skin test for eyelash tinting results in:

a) no change to the skin ○

b) the appearance of Vitiligo ○

c) irritation and even swelling in the area ○

d) the appearance of swollen eyes ○

Q11. A patch test should be carried out:

a) Seven days before the treatment date ○

b) 10 days before the treatment date ○

c) 24–48 hours before the treatment date ○

d) annually ○

Q12. What strength of hydrogen peroxide is mixed with eyelash tint?

a) 5 vol

b) 10 vol

c) 15 vol

d) 29 vol

Q13. Which one of the following comes under COSHH regulations?

a) hydrogen peroxide

b) eye make-up remover

c) petroleum jelly

d) liquid eye make-up remover

Q14. A *negative* reaction to a patch test means:

a) another patch test should be carried out

b) the client is unsuitable for treatment

c) the client must sign an indemnity form

d) the client is suitable for treatment

Q15. Lash and brow tint contains:

a) toluenediamine

b) peroxide

c) potassium hydroxide

d) humectants

Q16. The processing time for eyelash tinting on a natural redhead is?

a) the same as on any other client

b) shorter because the hair processes quickly

c) longer because the hair is resistant

d) accelerated as red hair is more absorbent

Q17. Conjunctivitis is a condition which is:

a) not infectious

b) caused by a virus

c) highly infectious

d) caused by a patch test

Q18. Which of the following would contra-indicate a lash and brow tint?

a) asthma ◯

b) stye ◯

c) nervous clients ◯

d) contact lens wearers ◯

Q19. Individual false eyelashes, if properly applied and cared for, can last up to:

a) one week ◯

b) two weeks ◯

c) three weeks ◯

d) four weeks ◯

Q20. Individual false lashes are removed by lifting them gently from the eye with:

a) sterile tweezers ◯

b) eye make-up remover ◯

c) cleansing lotion ◯

d) solvent ◯

MULTIPLE CHOICE TEST – ANSWERS

1.	A	6.	A	11.	C	16.	C
2.	C	7.	D	12.	B	17.	C
3.	B	8.	B	13.	A	18.	B
4.	A	9.	B	14.	D	19.	D
5.	C	10.	C	15.	A	20.	D

Marking and Grading

All correct   fantastic

One or two errors   excellent, well done

15 correct   very good, revise a bit more to improve your mark

12 correct   borderline pass: you need to revise a bit more so you go into a test with more confidence. You can do it!

Below 12   Go back to your revision notes and Revision Maps and spend a bit more time revising; then have another attempt

FINAL END TEST

This section consists of statements. Each one may be correct or incorrect. The answer required is simply

Yes or No.

In your assessment of whether the statement is correct or incorrect, you must only base your answer on the information provided. The questions are arranged in groups in the order that the related topics occurred in the text. After ensuring that all the questions have been answered, check the answers yourself on page 242.

• FINAL END TEST

1. Automatic tweezers are useful for clients who find eyebrow shaping very painful.

2. Poor quality tweezers can rust if immersed in sterilising fluid regularly.

3. The face shape and the natural shape of the eyebrow are important when determining the finished eyebrow shape.

4. Face shapes should *not* be considered during eyebrow shaping treatments.

5. An eyebrow reshape costs the same as an eyebrow trim.

6. Long untidy eyebrows can age a mature client.

7. On very strong eyebrow hairs, facial steaming could be incorporated into the treatment to open the pores.

8. Cold compresses should be applied during eyebrow shaping treatments to keep the follicle open.

9. Surgical spirit is never used in the eye area.

10. A mild antiseptic solution should be chosen to wipe over the area on completion of the shaping treatment.

11. A successful eyebrow shaping treatment will emphasise the client's eyes and be suitable for the client's age.

12. A stye and conjunctivitis would contra-indicate an eyebrow shape.

13. Lash tinting treatments are an excellent recommendation for contact lens and glasses wearers.

14. People who wear contact lenses cannot have eyelash tinting.

15. Many lash-tinting customers book a treatment before a holiday.

16. A *negative* reaction to a patch test means there is no reaction and the treatment can go ahead.

17. A *positive* reaction to a skin test means there is a skin reaction probably with irritation or redness. The treatment can not go ahead.

18. Any available peroxide can be mixed with eyelash tint.

19. Hydrogen peroxide comes under COSHH regulations because it is an irritant.

20. Only 10 vol peroxide is used in lash and brow tinting treatments.

21. Full details of any patch testing carried out must be carefully documented on the client record card.

22. A stye is a bacterial infection of the sebaceous gland of an eyelash.

23. Conjunctivitis is a bacterial infection that affects the mucous membrane that covers the eye and the eyelid.

24. Shaping is always carried out on *completion* of any lash and brow tinting.

25. One of the reasons why clients with eczema in the eye area are contra-indicated to tinting is because the skin is often broken and tint could enter.

26. Extra time may need to be allocated when booking an eyelash tint on a natural redhead.

27. Strip lashes can last for two weeks if cared for properly.

28. Individual lashes can last up to four weeks if properly cared for.

29. Strip lashes are normally applied to the client on completion of the make-up application.

30. A skin test should be carried out 24–48 hours prior to lash application to ascertain if the client could be allergic to the adhesive.

FINAL END TEST **ANSWERS**

1. Yes
2. Yes
3. Yes
4. No   The client's face shape should be considered when advising and providing eyebrow shaping treatments.
5. No   More would be charged to reshape the eyebrows, as more time would be allocated.
6. Yes
7. Yes
8. No   Cold compresses would close the follicle.
9. Yes
10. Yes
11. Yes
12. Yes
13. Yes
14. No   Contact lens wearers are frequent customers for this treatment. However, the lenses should be removed during treatment.
15. Yes
16. Yes
17. Yes
18. No   Only 10 vol peroxide is safe for use.
19. Yes
20. Yes
21. Yes
22. Yes
23. Yes
24. Yes
25. Yes
26. Yes
27. No   Strip lashes are not for long term use. They are for a 'single event' eg fashion show, special occasion.
28. Yes
29. Yes
30. Yes

Marking Guide and Grading

Check your answers and then check them against the guide below. In percentage terms 60% is considered a pass. With this type of end test, because it's a simple Yes or No answer, there is a strong likelihood you could have guessed some of the answers! You should take this into account when determining your grade.

Above 27 correct answers   is exceptional!

24 correct answers   a credit – excellent

18 correct answers   a pass – well done

Below 18 correct answers means you need to spend more time revising, so go back to your course notes and Revision Maps and then have another go.

CHECKLIST ✓ Can You?

MAKE-UP APPLICATION

When examiners prepare questions to test a candidate's knowledge of make-up, the questions have to be produced in such a way that it is fair to both the candidate and the person who is marking the answer; questions are often set around theoretical clients.

Because of this factor, you can expect corrective make-up and make-up questions to be based on general principles. These questions are not able to explore the colour-blending abilities and creativity of the candidate, they test the facts and basic principles of the theory of make-up application.

Corrective make-up is a popular subject for testing because it follows strict principles. It is easier for the examiner to ask direct meaningful questions about correcting an overlarge nose or a florid complexion, than to ask questions about a suitable make-up for a grandmother with silver hair!

REMEMBER!

Always remember the following make-up principles:

- Darker colours diminish, recede, or push back an area.
- Lighter colours emphasise, or bring forward an area.

Corrective make-up includes:

1. Concealing blemishes, age spots or pigmentation irregularities.
2. Enhancing a dull or florid skin colour.
3. Improving the appearance of puffy eyes and dark undereye circles.
4. Correcting creases such as the naso-labial folds.
5. Using highlighting and shading products to enhance good points and diminish poor points.
6. Using highlighting and shading products to balance face shapes and bone structure.
7. Using lip and eye cosmetics to enhance and balance the face.

Make sure that you have had some experience in attempting corrective make-up for the seven areas listed, so that you can write about it first-hand if a question should arise on a test paper.

Composition of make-up products

Candidates should expect questions to be prepared covering the likely *composition* and *ingredients* of the cosmetics we use. A general familiarity with product ingredients should stand you in good stead.

Use of make-up products

Candidates should expect questions around the correct use of cosmetic products. Popular areas for questioning include:

1. Choices of foundation for different skin types and skin colours.

2. Products to avoid if the skin is lined, eg:
   a) frosty foundations and powders
   b) frosty eye cosmetics.

3. Choosing make-up colour themes to match an outfit, eg *not* choosing a pink or mauve theme to match a peach or orange dress!

4. The requirements for producing an evening make-up, eg:
   a) stronger, darker eye colours
   b) brighter, stronger lip colours
   c) extra blusher, shader and highlighter
   d) a heavier, textured foundation.

5. The requirements for producing a bridal make-up, eg:
   a) subtle effect
   b) an effect that will photograph well (not all shiny)
   c) matching any flowers and the overall colour theme, harmonises with the gown, suit or outfit.

6. The requirements for producing a working day make-up, eg:
   a) totally natural effect
   b) matches the outfit to be worn
   c) lip and eye colours more soft and muted
   d) lighter textured foundation that looks natural in a working environment
   e) less blusher, shading products and mascara.

Revision Map – Contra-indications and the Make-up Treatment

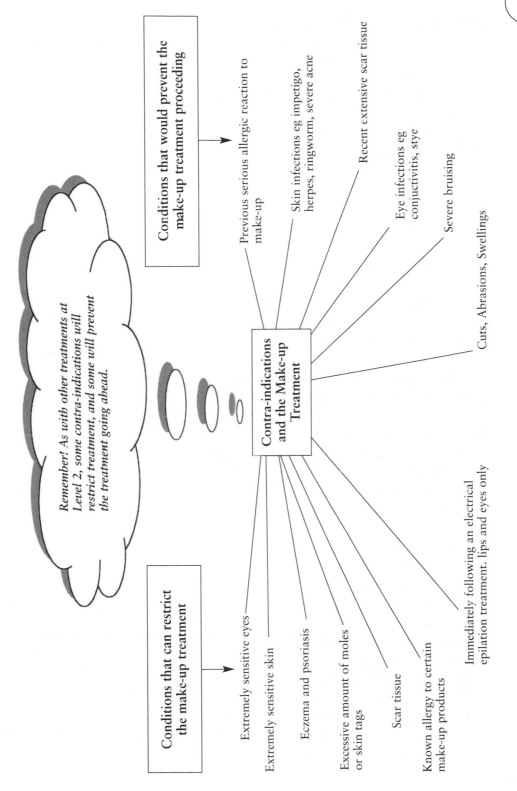

Remember! As with other treatments at Level 2, some contra-indications will restrict treatment, and some will prevent the treatment going ahead.

Conditions that would prevent the make-up treatment proceeding

Conditions that can restrict the make-up treatment

Contra-indications and the Make-up Treatment

Previous serious allergic reaction to make-up

Skin infections eg impetigo, herpes, ringworm, severe acne

Recent extensive scar tissue

Eye infections eg conjuctivitis, stye

Severe bruising

Cuts, Abrasions, Swellings

Immediately following an electrical epilation treatment. lips and eyes only

Known allergy to certain make-up products

Scar tissue

Excessive amount of moles or skin tags

Eczema and psoriasis

Extremely sensitive skin

Extremely sensitive eyes

Revision Map – Devising a Make-up Plan

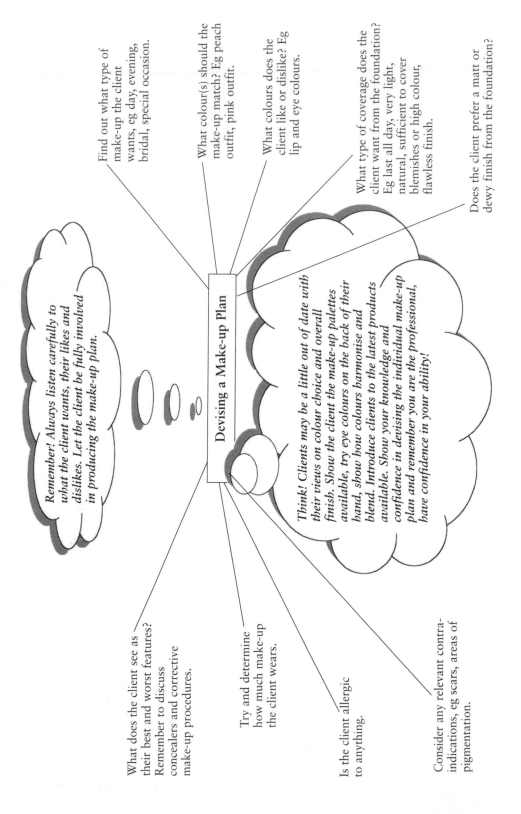

Find out what type of make-up the client wants, eg day, evening, bridal, special occasion.

What colour(s) should the make-up match? Eg peach outfit, pink outfit.

What colours does the client like or dislike? Eg lip and eye colours.

What type of coverage does the client want from the foundation? Eg last all day, very light, natural, sufficient to cover blemishes or high colour, flawless finish.

Does the client prefer a matt or dewy finish from the foundation?

Remember! Always listen carefully to what the client wants, their likes and dislikes. Let the client be fully involved in producing the make-up plan.

Devising a Make-up Plan

Think! Clients may be a little out of date with their views on colour choice and overall finish. Show the client the make-up palettes available, try eye colours on the back of their hand, show how colours harmonise and blend. Introduce clients to the latest products available. Show your knowledge and confidence in devising the individual make-up plan and remember you are the professional, have confidence in your ability!

What does the client see as their best and worst features? Remember to discuss concealers and corrective make-up procedures.

Try and determine how much make-up the client wears.

Is the client allergic to anything.

Consider any relevant contra-indications, eg scars, areas of pigmentation.

Revision Map A – Make-up Products

Concealers
- Mask minor imperfections.
- In various shades, including green, beige or white.
- Comes in stick, wand or pot form.
- Thicker concealers contain more pigment so have more coverage.

Remedial Camouflage Creams
- Thick cream based products with *very* dense pigments.
- Covers blemishes and birth marks completely.
- Set with a special fixing powder.
- Large range of colours and tones including white, yellow and grey.

Pre Make-up bases

Moisturisers
- Help maintain moisture levels and provide a good base for make-up.
- The right choice of moisturiser can add to the lasting properties of the make-up.

Colour Washes
- Bases which correct skin tone, eg green – reduces redness and florid skin; Mauve – brightens a dull, sallow skin.

Skin illuminators
- Imparts a warm iridescent glow.
- Aimed to imitate a youthful glow.
- Contains fine, densely-packed, glistening particles.
- Some have gold tones, some pink or beige.
- Many have SPF.

Make-up Primers
- Specially formulated, applied under moisturiser.
- Adds a tightening invisible veil to the surface layer of the skin.
- Greatly extends the lasting properties of the make-up, so useful for bridal work.
- Enhances the overall appearance of the skin.

Remember! Specialist treatment foundations are available from leading cosmetic companies with formulations that include UV screens, anti-pollution agents, lifting and firming properties and light reflecting agents. Foundation manufacture is always changing so pay a visit to your local department store.

MAP A
Make-up Products

Block or Cake Foundations
- Suitable for most skin.
- Compressed creams with the addition of powder and pigment.
- Applied with damp sponge.
- Coverage depends on application, generally medium to heavy.
- More popular for home use than salon use.

Foundations

Medicated
- Often water or alcohol based.
- For oily, problem skin.
- Often contains ingredients to promote healing and absorb excessive sebum.

Cream
- Excellent for dryer and mature skin.
- Oil based.
- Gives smooth, even coverage.
- Set with powder.

Liquid
- Generally contains less oil than cream foundations.
- Suitable for most skins.
- Provides a natural effect with medium coverage.

Gels
- A liquid tint with the addition of a gelling agent.
- Gives natural sun-kissed appearance.
- Effective on tanned and black skin.

Powder Creams or All-In-One
- Come in compact form.
- Perfect blend of powder and cream for good coverage without a mask-like appearance.
- Applied with a sponge.
- Suitable for most skin types.

Revision Map B – Make-up Products

**MAP B
Make-up Products**

Loose Powder

- Most powders contain talc for slip, mica for iridescence, magnesium carbonate for absorption, colour pigments and perfume.
- Used to set or fix the foundation.
- Translucent powders most popular as they don't alter the colour of the foundation.
- Lightweight powders give a natural effect.
- Heavier powders are less popular and add additional colour to the skin, giving a more 'made up' appearance.
- Always apply liberally and dust off excess in a downward motion.

Pressed Powder

- Contains the same ingredients with the addition of a gum, and is pressed into a compact form.
- Ideal for touching up a make-up application.
- Not fine enough to set a foundation application.

Blushers

- Used to give vitality to the face and enhance the eyes.
- Many formulations, gels, creams and powders.
- Similar in formulation to foundations and powder but with different colour pigments.
- Pinks, mauves, peaches, gingers and browns, matt and frosty.
- Colour choice should be dominated by the overall make-up theme.

Remember! Black skin needs stronger colours eg reds, oranges and deep mauves.

*Remember!
You must look at new products being sold by the leading cosmetic manufacturers. Every season new powders are developed to provide 'that season's look'. Have a look at the multicoloured beads and pressed powders on sale, that enhance skin tones and encourage reflection of light to give the skin a more youthful glow. They are good to work with and very effective.*

Revision Map C – Make-up Products

MAP C Make-up Products

Eyebrow Cosmetics
- Used to define the brows.
- Pencils, easy to use, similar to eyeshadow pencils but much harder.
- Powders, applied with a stiff brush, used wet or dry.
- The composition of eyebrow defining powders is similar to eyeshadows.

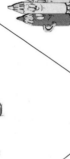

Eyeshadow
- Used to enhance the eyes.
- Available in different colours and forms, eg:

Powders
- Long lasting, compressed or loose, mica often included to give frosting.
- Basic ingredients: talc, oils and pigments.

Pencils and Crayons
- Easy to apply.
- Comprised of waxes, oils and colour pigments.

Creams
- Tend to crease, but useful on very dry skin.
- Contains oils, waxes and pigments.

Gels
- Adds gloss rather than colour.
- More popular with young clientele.

Eyeliner
- Used for defining eye shape and accentuating the lashes.
- Eyeliner looks more natural if it matches the eyeshadow colour.

Liquid Liner
- Applied with a fine sable brush.
- Oil in water or gum solution with pigments.

Cake Liner
- Applied with a fine wet brush.
- Easier to control, similar in composition to powder eyeshadows.

Pencils or Crayons
- Easy to apply.
- Available in many colours, contains waxes, oils and colour pigments.

Mascara
- Used to colour, thicken and darken the lashes.
- Available in many colours including fashion colours.
- Some formulas contain silk particles that build up lashes or proteins to condition the lashes, some formulas are waterproof. Common ingredient is petroleum jelly.
- Cream mascara is a water in oil emulsion, easy to remove.
- Liquid mascara, popular, contains castor oil and synthetic resins.
- Special inorganic pigments are used to give colour without irritating the eye.
- Block mascara, very economical and more hygienic in use, but surpassed by the fantastic formulations now available.

Fun colours!
Try blue mascara on dark eyes violet on green eyes, turquoise on grey or blue eyes, green on brown eyes.

Revision Map D – Make-up Products

Highlighters and Shaders
- Similar in composition to blusher but with different pigments.
- True highlighting and shading products more popular in photographic work.
- Very effective if applied correctly.
- Available in powders, creams and sticks.

Remember! Lip cosmetics should harmonise the total make-up effect. Common ingredients are: petroleum jelly, lanolin, beeswax, carnuba wax, silicone, castor oil, preservative, colourants, mica for frosty effect.

Lip Pencils
- Less oil content, harder.
- Used to outline the lips.
- Prevents lip colour bleeding.

MAP D
Make-up Products

Lipstick
- High wax content which helps form lipstick shape.
- Has emollients, oils like castor oil to soften and lubricate lips.
- Sun block or UV screen.
- Organic pigments used to colour without staining.
- Some contain fragrance.
- Many colours available.

Lip Gloss
- Clear or coloured.
- Gives a 'wet look' shine.
- Contains mineral oils and bentonite clay.
- Natural appearance.

*Question –
Why do lipsticks bleed?*
- No lipliner used to outline lips.
- Lines around mouth encourage seepage.
- High oil content which when the body temperature warms it.

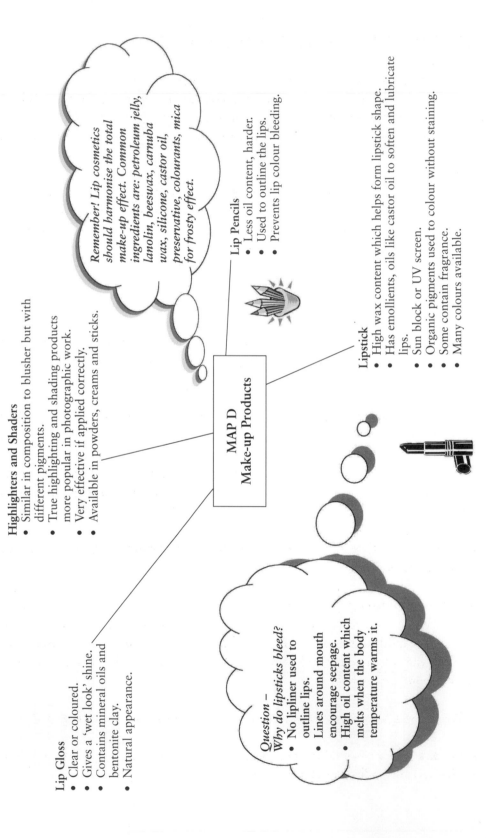

Review your course notes, text books and client record cards.
Study the Revision Maps provided for you and examples of multiple choice
and short answer questions. When you feel comfortable and familiar with the
chapter contents, have a go at the multiple choice end test and the final end test.

Note:
*Information you should know about skin structure and anatomy and
physiology will not be featured in this chapter. Some of the questions included
in this chapter will include aspects of skin structure, anatomy and hygiene
already covered in Chapters 1, 3 and 4.*

SHORT ANSWER QUESTIONS

Examples of short answer and multiple choice questions around the previous
Revision Maps are provided for you. Reviewing them should assist your
revision process.

Q1. Why is pressed powder never used to set the foundation in a professional
make-up application? *(2 marks)*

Answer: Pressed powder is not fine enough in its composition to set the foundation
application. It also contains a gum which could interfere with the chemistry of the
foundation.

Q2. Briefly outline the differences between a lightweight loose powder and a
heavy loose powder. *(4 marks)*

Answer: Lightweight powders set the make-up base effectively but have a natural
finish. Heavy loose powders also effectively set the make-up base, but they impart a
less natural finish to the end result. These powders often contain more colour pigments
and can add colour to the make-up base which, unless carefully chosen, can result in a
patchy foundation finish.

Q3. Why is blusher used in a make-up application treatment? *(3 marks)*

Answer: Blusher is used to enhance the eyes and give vitality to the face. It is also
needed to balance the overall make-up.

Q4. Why is impetigo a contra-indication to a make-up application treatment?

(3 marks)

Answer: Impetigo is a bacterial infection which is highly contagious. This condition could be extended and worsened by a make-up treatment, and could be easily transmitted to the operator or other clients.

Q5. When should the therapist ascertain if the client has any known allergies to make-up? Justify your answer. *(5 marks)*

Answer: During the client consultation.

The client consultation provides the therapist and client with the opportunity to ask and answer questions. A professional therapist must always ask if a client has any known allergies, so that any products that could cause the client to experience a reaction can be omitted from the treatment, or an alternative product sought.

Q6 (a). Why does the presence of eczema and psoriasis restrict, or even prevent, a make-up application treatment when both conditions are not contagious? *(5 marks)*

Answer: The preparation required prior to make-up application, namely cleansing, toning and moisturising, could irritate areas of eczema and psoriasis.

Make up products and cosmetics contain synthetic ingredients, colourings and preservatives which could easily irritate further the areas of skin affected by eczema and psoriasis.

Q6 (b). Give an example of the appearance of an eczema or psoriasis condition which would prevent treatment proceeding. *(2 marks)*

Answer: Treatment must not take place if the affected area is sensitive and the skin is broken or showing signs of infection.

Q6 (c). Give an example of the appearance of an eczema or psoriasis condition that could restrict but not prevent a make-up treatment. *(2 marks)*

Answer: Treatment can be restricted if the area is small enough to miss out without spoiling the effect of the make-up. The area should also be withheld from the cleansing routine.

Q7. Why must the lids and caps of make-up containers be replaced immediately after use?   *(1 mark)*

Answer: This is a hygiene requirement. Make-up containers and their contents could become infected by micro-organisms if they are not sealed after use.

Q8. Why are disposable make-up brushes and applicators preferred for salon use?   *(2 marks)*

Answer: The use of these items contributes towards optimum hygiene practices. These items require no cleaning and disinfecting, and are simply discarded after use.

Q9. How do hypoallergenic make-up products differ from standard make-up products?   *(2 marks)*

Answer: These products contain less preservatives, colour pigments, perfume amd other known irritants than standard ranges.

Q10. State two factors that help determine the colour choice for blusher products in the make-up sequence.   *(2 marks)*

Answer:
• The product used must match and enhance the overall colour theme of the make-up.
• The product used should not clash with the client's hair colouring, or the garment to be worn by the client.

Q11. How do lip pencils differ from lipsticks?   *(5 marks)*

Answer: Lip pencils differ in use and manufacture.

They are used to outline the lips and thus prevent lip colours bleeding into the surrounding skin. They are harder in composition and contain fewer oils than lipsticks.

Lipsticks are used to colour the lips and harmonise the total make-up effect. They contain oils, waxes and emollients that lubricate and condition the lips whilst adding colour to the face.

Q12. State the similarities and differences between the make-up products known as highlighters and shaders.   *(6 marks)*

Answer: *Similarities:*

• These products are similar in composition to blusher, but contain different colour pigments.

• Both highlighters and shaders are available in powders, creams and sticks.

• These products have a similar price point.

Differences:

• The products are used in an entirely different way, ie highlighters are used to enhance or bring forward good features, whereas shaders are used to diminish or recede over prominent features.

• The colours of highlighters include, ivory, bone, white, cream, soft beige, peach.

• The colours of shaders include all shades of browns, rusts and grey.

Q13. How can the make-up artist reduce the risks of lipcolours seeping into the skin around the mouth? Give five guidelines. *(5 marks)*

Answer:

• Use a specialist product on the lips known as lipstick primer.

• Apply a thin layer of foundation and loose powder over the lips.

• Outline the lips with a lip pencil.

• Blot the first application of lipstick with a tissue, and then re-apply a second layer of colour.

• Apply a thin layer of specialist lipcoating product which contains a small amount of spirit gum.

Note:

In this type of scenario, the make-up artist or therapist would be well advised to choose a harder type of lipstick, or certainly one which appeared less creamy in texture.

Q14. What actions should be taken if the client experiences itching and burning during the application of eye make-up? *(4 marks)*

Answer:

• The treatment must stop immediately.

• The eye cosmetics should be swiftly removed with eye make-up remover.

• Eye pads of dampened cotton wool soaked in water or witch hazel should be applied to the eyes to cool and soothe them.

• The contra-action should be fully detailed on the client record card.

Q15. Name four substances commonly used in the cosmetics industry which are known to cause adverse reactions in susceptible people. *(4 marks)*

Answer:
- Lanolin.
- Perfumes.
- Pearlising agents eg mica.
- Paraben.

(Other acceptable answers could include eosin, mineral oils, binding ingredients such as gums, and alcohols found in astringents.)

MULTIPLE CHOICE QUESTIONS

Some examples of multiple choice examination questions are included for you to enable you to give yourself a short test. Carefully consider the descriptions provided before choosing your answer. Only one answer is correct. Indicate your answer by putting an **X** in the circle: ◯.

Q1. Impetigo is a contra-indication to make-up application because:

a) it is non-contagious ◯

b) it is contagious ◯

c) it cannot be improved by make-up application ◯

d) it can be irritated by the application of make-up ◯

Q2. A client with sensitive eyes can undergo a make-up treatment providing:

a) hypoallergenic eye cosmetics are used ◯

b) mascara is omitted ◯

c) the eye area is excluded from the treatment ◯

d) frosted eye colours are not used ◯

Q3. Client make-up preferences and requirements should be ascertained:

a) by the receptionist when the appointment is made ◯

b) as the treatment is in progress ◯

c) by reading details of previous treatments ◯

d) during the client consultation ◯

Q4. If a client has a receding chin, the receding bone would be the:

a) maxilla ◯

b) mandible ◯

c) zygomatic ◯

d) temporal ◯

Q5. The bones that contribute to high cheekbones are the:

a) occipital bones ◯

b) nasal bones ◯

c) zygomatic bones ◯

d) maxillae ◯

Q6. A client with a high forehead has a large:

a) parietal bone ◯

b) mandible ◯

c) occipital bone ◯

d) frontal bone ◯

Q7. Which one of the following foundations imparts a healthy glow effect on the skin?

a) liquid foundation ◯

b) cream foundation ◯

c) powder cream foundation ◯

d) gel foundation ◯

Q8. Which one of the following foundations would be the *best choice* for a dry, mature skin condition?

a) A medicated foundation with SPF ◯

b) A liquid foundation with SPF ◯

c) A cream foundation with SPF ◯

d) A gel foundation with SPF ◯

Q9. A common ingredient in loose face powder is:

a) kaolin ○

b) gum ○

c) beeswax ○

d) magnesium carbonate ○

Q10. Which *one* of the following produces a 'frosty' effect in eyeshadows and lipsticks?

a) mica ○

b) petroleum jelly ○

c) carnuba wax ○

d) the colour pigments ○

Q11. Organic pigments are used in lipstick manufacture because they:

a) stain the lips ○

b) do not stain the lips ○

c) have emollient properties ○

d) have a light fragrance ○

Q12. What is the main purpose of mascara?

a) to colour and thicken the lashes ○

b) to even up irregular eye shapes ○

c) to bring out the eyebrow shape ○

d) to enhance the client's eyes in-between eyelash tinting treatments ○

Q13. Which one of the following would be the *best* foundation choice for an oily problem skin type?

a) cream ○

b) gel ○

c) powder cream ○

d) medicated ○

Q14. The ingredient eosin is a red pigment which can cause adverse reactions in some individuals. In what product is eosin found?

a) shading products ◯

b) eyeshadow ◯

c) lipstick ◯

d) foundation ◯

Q15. Lanolin is a substance similar to sebum. It is used as a softening ingredient in products such as hand creams and moisturisers. Lanolin can cause adverse reactions in some individuals. From which animal is lanolin produced?

a) sheep ◯

b) goats ◯

c) cows ◯

d) bulls ◯

Q16. Paraben is used in the cosmetics industry. It can cause adverse reactions in some individuals. What type of product is paraben?

a) a perfume ◯

b) a preservative ◯

c) a binding ingredient ◯

d) a colourant ◯

Q17. Which one of the following is a contra-indication to make-up application?

a) the wearing of contact lenses ◯

b) an area of vitiligo ◯

c) ringworm ◯

d) a port wine stain ◯

Q18. Which one of the following is contagious?

a) conjunctivitis ○

b) eczema ○

c) hypersensitive eyes ○

d) leucoderma ○

Q19. Which one of the following is *not* a contra-indication to make-up application?

a) impetigo ○

b) lentigo ○

c) herpes simplex ○

d) severe bruising ○

Q20. When applying lipcolour to a client with deep vertical lines around the mouth, what should the therapist use?

a) lip gloss ○

b) rich creamy lipstick ○

c) lipliner to outline the lips ○

d) lip brush ○

MULTIPLE CHOICE TEST – ANSWERS

1.	B	6.	D	11.	B	16.	B
2.	A	7.	D	12.	A	17.	C
3.	D	8.	C	13.	D	18.	A
4.	B	9.	D	14.	C	19.	B
5.	C	10.	A	15.	A	20.	C

Marking and Grading

17 correct   a credit, excellent

13 correct   a pass, well done

Just below 10   you're nearly there. Keep revising, review the Revision Maps and have another go

Below 5   you need to spend more time revising. Look again at your course notes and the Revision Maps, and have another go in a week's time.

Revision Map – Corrective Make-up
Face Shapes 1

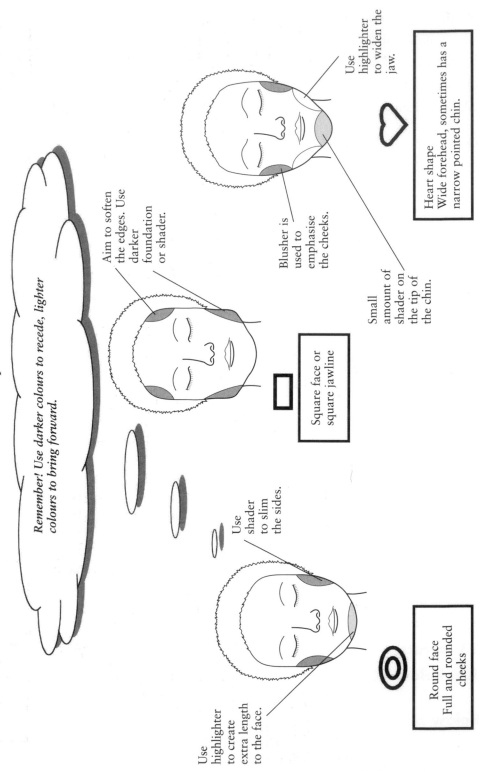

Remember! Use darker colours to recede, lighter colours to bring forward.

Aim to soften the edges. Use darker foundation or shader.

Square face or square jawline

Blusher is used to emphasise the cheeks.

Small amount of shader on the tip of the chin.

Use highlighter to widen the jaw.

Heart shape
Wide forehead, sometimes has a narrow pointed chin.

Use highlighter to create extra length to the face.

Use shader to slim the sides.

Round face
Full and rounded cheeks

Revision Map – Corrective Make-up
Face Shapes 2

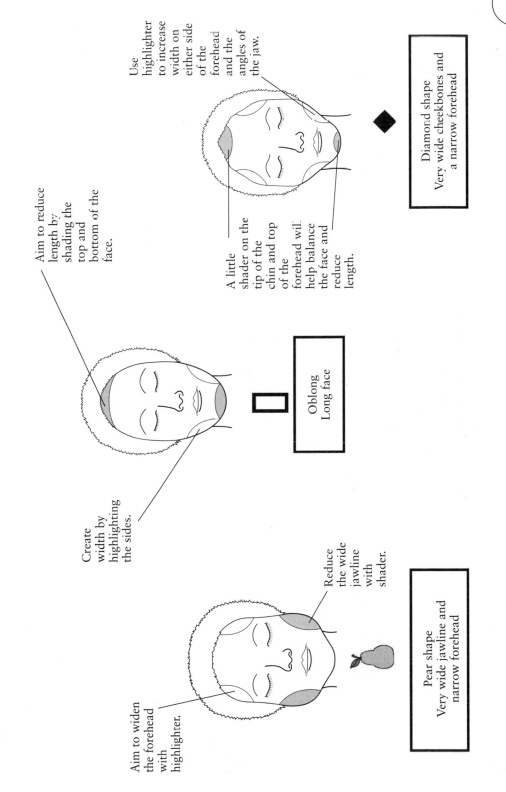

Aim to reduce length by shading the top and bottom of the face.

Create width by highlighting the sides.

Oblong
Long face

Use highlighter to increase width on either side of the forehead and the angles of the jaw.

A little shader on the tip of the chin and top of the forehead will help balance the face and reduce length.

Diamond shape
Very wide cheekbones and a narrow forehead

Reduce the wide jawline with shader.

Aim to widen the forehead with highlighter.

Pear shape
Very wide jawline and narrow forehead

Revision Map – Corrective Make-up
Common Considerations – Eyes

Eyes too close together
- Use light colours only on the inner eye area.
- Try and lift the eye with a gentle arch to the eyebrow.
- Use highlighter under the brow.
- On the outer corners, use darker eye colours.

Eyes too wide apart
- Use darker colours only on the inner eye area.
- Use lighter colours only on the outer eye area.

Protruding eyes
- Use darker colours carefully blended over the eyelid.
- Use a small amount of highlighter on the browbone only.
- Always avoid a round eyebrow shape.

Puffy eyes
- Causes creases below areas of puffy tissue.
- Use cooling eye gels.
- Minimise the baggy puffy area with a slightly darker foundation.
- Use a lighter foundation on the creased area underneath the 'bags'.

Eyes

The client wears glasses
- Always look at the lenses. Some lenses make the eyes bigger, some smaller.
- In general, heavy frames call for a stronger make-up.
- Use muted eye colours on bright frames.
- Use soft colours with lightweight metal frames.
- Always use eyebrow pencil and mascara carefully on glasses wearers to define the eyes subtly.

Deep set eyes
- Use pale, preferably frosty colours to bring the eyes forward, apply all over.
- Apply a darker colour along the socket line, carefully blended.
- Use lots of mascara.

Dark under eye circles
- Use specialist light, white or slightly tinted concealing products underneath the make-up.
- Use a lighter foundation if no concealing product is available.
- Do not overdo it.

Remember! By using the principles of highlight and shade, most eye shapes can be enhanced. Always consider a side and frontal view when making up the eyes, stand back and have a look at your work from a distance. Consider how the eyes balance with the rest of the client's features.

Revision Map – Corrective Make-up
Common Considerations – Lips and Noses

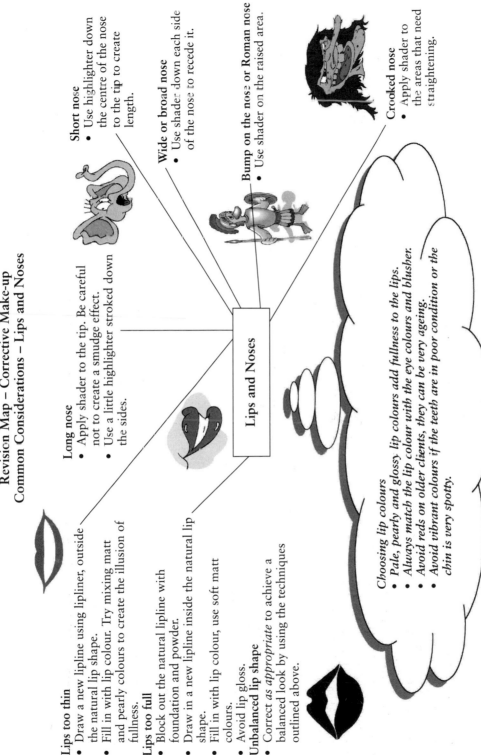

Short nose
- Use highlighter down the centre of the nose to the tip to create length.

Wide or broad nose
- Use shader down each side of the nose to recede it.

Bump on the nose or Roman nose
- Use shader on the raised area.

Crooked nose
- Apply shader to the areas that need straightening.

Long nose
- Apply shader to the tip. Be careful not to create a smudge effect.
- Use a little highlighter stroked down the sides.

Lips and Noses

Lips too thin
- Draw a new lipline using lipliner, outside the natural lip shape.
- Fill in with lip colour. Try mixing matt and pearly colours to create the illusion of fullness.

Lips too full
- Block out the natural lipline with foundation and powder.
- Draw in a new lipline inside the natural lip shape.
- Fill in with lip colour, use soft matt colours.
- Avoid lip gloss.

Unbalanced lip shape
- Correct *as appropriate* to achieve a balanced look by using the techniques outlined above.

Choosing lip colours
- *Pale, pearly and glossy lip colours add fullness to the lips.*
- *Always match the lip colour with the eye colours and blusher.*
- *Avoid reds on older clients, they can be very ageing.*
- *Avoid vibrant colours if the teeth are in poor condition or the chin is very spotty.*

Revision Map – Corrective Make-up
General Points

General Points

Naso-labial folds
- Caused through relaxation of musculature.
- Deep creases running from the nose to the edges of the mouth.
- Use a light foundation or cover stick on the darkest area.
- Carefully blend normal foundation on top.

Florid or red complexions
- Could be through broken blood capillaries or merely through general skin colour.
- Use a green corrective moisturiser.
- Use beige foundations, medium to high coverage. Avoid any foundations with pink or peach tones.

Dull sallow complexions
- Can be through age or oiliness.
- Can be brightened up with a mauve colour wash.
- Avoid foundations with yellow tones.
- Use foundations with beige or slightly rose tones.

Pigmentation patches
- Dark patchy areas of brown pigmentation common on mature skin.
- Cover with a masking cream or thick concealer prior to foundation application.

Perspiration
- Excessive perspiration and a warm skin temperature can make application of make-up difficult.
- Keep the client as cool as possible.
- Blot perspiration with a soft tissue.
- Occasionally spray the face with a fine mineral water spray.
- Work as quickly as possible.
- Choose foundations with a high water content.

Double chin and jowls
- Caused through loss of muscular tone.
- Apply shader to the offending area.
- Blend it in well.

Sensitive skin
- As far as possible, use hypoallergenic products.

CORRECTIVE MAKE-UP

Look at your course work notes and the Revision Maps on pages 262–266 around the main aspects of corrective make-up. Review the sample multiple choice and short answer questions provided for you around this topic.

SHORT ANSWER QUESTIONS

Q1. State two features of the product known as concealing cream.   *(2 marks)*

Answer: Concealing cream is a thick concealer. It contains more pigments than liquids, wands or sticks.

Q2. What foundation can be recommended for a client with post acne scarring?   *(2 marks)*

Answer: A covering foundation should be recommended, possibly a powder cream type or a block foundation which would offer good coverage with easy application using a cosmetic sponge.

Q3. State two make-up type products a client could use to minimise a florid skin condition.   *(1 mark)*

Answer:
• A green tinted moisturiser or colour wash.
• A flat beige foundation.

Q4. How can the therapist slim down a round face shape during a make-up treatment?   *(2 marks)*

Answer: A round face shape can be slimmed down by applying shader or a darker foundation product to the sides of the face. Highlighter could be applied to the chin to create the illusion of extra length to the face.

Q5. Describe the features of a diamond face shape, and outline how this face shape could be improved by highlighting and shading techniques.   *(5 marks)*

Answer: A diamond face shape has a narrow forehead and very wide cheekbones. The face can appear quite sharp and angular.

Highlighting products should be used to increase the width of the face just above the temples, and at the angles of the jaw.

A small amount of shading product should be used on the tip of the chin and the top of the forehead to reduce the length of the face and balance with the sides. Obviously, if the client wears a fringe, the shading on the forehead should be omitted.

Q6. What type of eyebrow shape *must* be avoided with a round face shape?

(1 mark)

Answer: A rounded eyebrow shape must be avoided.

The following four questions refer to the text below.

Lucy has an oily complexion with a dull sallow appearance. She complains her eyes are too close together and her nose is too short. Lucy has booked for a cleanse and make-up treatment.

Q7. Which products should be used on this client underneath the foundation application?

(2 marks)

Answer: A light moisturiser or oil absorbing moisturiser should be used on this client. A mauve or violet liquid colourwash should be used to correct the sallow, dull skin appearance.

Q8. How can the eyes be made to appear less close together?

(3 marks)

Answer: By using light colours on the inner eye area and a darker shade on the outer corners of the eyes, the eyes can be made to appear less close. A light highlighter can be used just below the eyebrow, and the eyebrow hairs brushed or shaped into a gentle arch.

Q9. State the corrective make-up technique which can be used to lengthen a short nose.

(2 marks)

Answer: Length can be created by applying a highlighter to the centre of the nose from the bridge to the nose tip.

Q10. What is the maximum acceptable treatment time to carry out this simple corrective make-up suitable for day wear, with a basic cleanse, tone, moisturise and proper client consultation? *(1 mark)*

Answer: No longer than 40 minutes.

Q11. Outline how the appearance of a double chin condition can be minimised during a corrective make-up session. *(2 marks)*

Answer: A shading product or darker foundation can be applied to the area and carefully blended in. This will help recede the double chin condition.

Q12. Name three muscles which contribute to the appearance of a double chin and jowls. *(3 marks)*

Answer:
- Platysma.
- Depressors of the lower lip.
- Masseter.

Q13. Outline corrective make-up techniques that can be used to reduce the size of an overlarge mouth. *(4 marks)*

Answer:
1. Blot out the lips with the application of foundation and powder.
2. Draw in a new lip line inside the natural lip line with a lip pencil.
3. Apply a soft matt lip colour, blot with tissue, and reapply. Do not apply lip gloss.
4. Check the finished result balances with the eye make-up and the overall effect.

Q14. How can dark undereye circles be diminished prior to make-up? *(4 marks)*

Answer: A small amount of a lightweight concealer can be applied to this area using fingertips or a soft make-up brush. The colour chosen should be light enough to cover the dark circles, but be in harmony with the client's skin tone. Foundation and powder are then applied.

Q15. Outline the procedure for minimising the appearance of a heavy mandible. *(4 marks)*

Answer: A shading product can be stroked along the mandible or jawbone; alternatively, a darker shade of foundation could be used. The balance must be carefully checked and viewed from both front and side angles. It may be necessary to apply a small amount of highlighter in the centre of the jawbone and onto the neck, to give a more natural appearance.

Q16. a) Outline the recognition factors of the skin condition known as lentigo. *(3 marks)*
b) State how a small area of lentigo on the face could be concealed. *(2 marks)*

Answer:
a) Lentigo is a brown discoloration of the skin caused by areas of pigmentation. The colour of lentigo varies from individual to individual, and can range from light to dark brown. Lentigo can appear anywhere on the face or body, and can affect small or large areas.
b) A small area of lentigo on the face could be concealed by the application of a thick concealer and a medium to high coverage foundation.

MULTIPLE CHOICE QUESTIONS

Some examples of multiple choice examination questions are included for you to enable you to give yourself a short test. Carefully consider the descriptions provided before choosing your answer. Only one answer is correct. Indicate your answer by putting an **X** in the circle: ◯

Q1. To shorten an oblong or long face shape, shader should be applied to:
a) the hollow of the cheeks ◯
b) the tip of the chin and top of the forehead ◯
c) the angles of the jawbone ◯
d) the cheek bones ◯

Q2. Which of the following best describes the term a contra-action to make-up?

a) when the client is unsuitable for treatment ◯

b) when the client dislikes the finished result ◯

c) when the treatment has to be interrupted due to a reaction of some kind ◯

d) when the treatment has to be stopped and the client referred to their GP ◯

Q3. To reduce an overlarge lip shape, a suitable colour from the following list would be:

a) red matt ◯

b) magenta gloss ◯

c) bronze matt ◯

d) pale pink pearlised ◯

Q4. The best way to minimise overhanging eyelids is to:

a) shade the fullest part with a darker colour, and lift the eyebrows by using a slightly pearlised highlighter below the brow bone ◯

b) apply a mid-tone pearlised colour to the fullest part, and a light pearlised highlighter to the brow bone ◯

c) apply a light textured concealer to the eyelids, a thin eyeliner, and lashings of mascara ◯

d) highlight the fullest part with a light matt colour, and apply a darker eyeshadow to the area immediately above the lashes ◯

Q5. Vitiligo is caused by:

a) too much of the skin pigment melanin ◯

b) pregnancy ◯

c) total lack of the skin pigment melanin ◯

d) too little of the skin pigment melanin ◯

Q6. The procedure for improving a receding chin is to:

a) apply stronger, brighter lip colours ○

b) apply highlighter to the centre of the chin ○

c) apply shader to the centre of the chin ○

d) extend the blusher application to draw attention away from the chin ○

Q7. An appropriate corrective foundation for a pink skin tone would be:

a) golden toned ○

b) ivory toned ○

c) rose toned ○

d) beige toned ○

Q8. Camouflage creams differ from cover sticks because they:

a) are very dense and cover blemishes and birthmarks completely ○

b) are medicated ○

c) are set with damp cotton wool pads ○

d) are easier to remove ○

Q9. A suitable corrective technique to improve the appearance of a broad nose is to apply:

a) shader to each side of the bridge of the nose ○

b) shader to the sides of the nose ○

c) highlighter to the sides of the nose ○

d) shader to the tip of the nose ○

The following three questions refer to the text below:

Mrs Ruiz has a Mediterranean background, an olive skin tone, and a layer of fine, dark facial hair on the upper lip and sides of the face. The eyes are dark and oval, and the client's lip shape is even. Her outfit is orange.

Q10. Which of the following products could be used to enhance the client's skin tone without emphasising the facial hair?

a) loose face powder ○

b) a cream foundation ○

c) a fine layer of pressed bronzing powder ○

d) an all-in-one foundation ○

Q11. The main emphasis of the make-up application for this client is to:

a) enhance the lips and eyes ○

b) disguise the facial hair ○

c) even out the colour of the skin ○

d) distract attention from the eyes ○

Q12. An *unsuitable* lipcolour would be:

a) peach ○

b) bronze ○

c) ginger ○

d) cerise ○

MULTIPLE CHOICE TEST – ANSWERS

1.	B	4.	A	7.	D	10.	C
2.	C	5.	C	8.	A	11.	A
3.	C	6.	B	9.	B	12.	D

Marking and Grading

10 correct a credit, excellent

8 correct a pass, well done

Just below 7 you're nearly there. Keep revising, review the Revision Maps and have another go

Below 4 you need to spend more time revising. Look again at your course notes and the Revision Maps, and have another go in a week's time.

DEVISING TREATMENT PLANS

You should be able to accomplish this task quite naturally and regularly in practical sessions. Sometimes your ability to do this is tested by providing you with scenarios, which describe a client and ask you to choose a treatment plan from examples provided. Only *one* treatment plan is correct, and the other treatment plans should be eliminated. Sometimes it is easy to perform the elimination process because the treatment plans are quite clearly wrong; at other times it is more difficult because the differences between plans are more subtle.

There are two things to be done when answering scenario type questions:
1. Look carefully, point by point, at the description of the client. Carefully consider what is required by the client, ask yourself, 'What are the client's needs?'
2. Systematically look at each stage of the treatment plan and judge for yourself – *Yes*, this would meet the clients needs and is appropriate; or *No*, this is not needed and is not appropriate.

An example of a client scenario and possible treatment plans is provided for you. You will see that an attempt has been made to fit each step of the treatment plan against the client's requirements. By doing this it is easier to arrive at the correct answer.

Sample Treatment Plans

Question: Select the most appropriate plan for Mrs Price.

Answer: Plan C

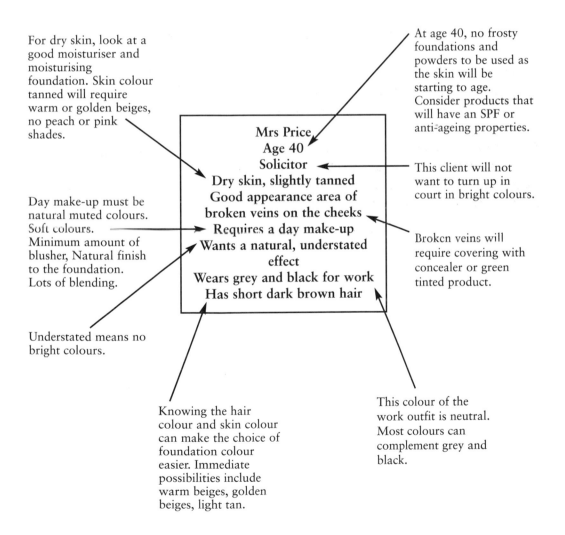

By carefully looking point by point at
the description of the client we can
actually determine her treatment needs.

For dry skin, look at a good moisturiser and moisturising foundation. Skin colour tanned will require warm or golden beiges, no peach or pink shades.

At age 40, no frosty foundations and powders to be used as the skin will be starting to age. Consider products that will have an SPF or anti-ageing properties.

Mrs Price
Age 40
Solicitor
Dry skin, slightly tanned
Good appearance area of
broken veins on the cheeks
Requires a day make-up
Wants a natural, understated
effect
Wears grey and black for work
Has short dark brown hair

This client will not want to turn up in court in bright colours.

Day make-up must be natural muted colours. Soft colours. Minimum amount of blusher, Natural finish to the foundation. Lots of blending.

Broken veins will require covering with concealer or green tinted product.

Understated means no bright colours.

Knowing the hair colour and skin colour can make the choice of foundation colour easier. Immediate possibilities include warm beiges, golden beiges, light tan.

This colour of the work outfit is neutral. Most colours can complement grey and black.

PLAN A

- Liquid moisturiser.
- Application of all-in-one powder cream foundation, light beige.
- Application of loose face powder.
- Light application of black mascara.
- Dusting of blusher in warm peach.
- Matt lipstick in Peach Ginger.

Yes – this plan offers appealing peachy lip colours and blusher but no eyeshadow, so the result could look unbalanced.

Also, the client wants a natural understated look. Powder cream foundation has a medium to heavy coverage, plus an application of loose powder would produce a 'make up' finish which the client has not requested.

Yes – the black mascara would be suitable; it would tone in with the client's hair and match the outfit to be worn.

REJECTED!
Think! This plan can be improved

PLAN B

- Moisturiser with SPF8.
- Specialist lifting foundation in Natural Light Tan.
- Ivory highlighter and mid-Grape eyeshadow to the eyes.
- Soft grey mascara.
- Dusting of mid pink blusher.
- Matt lipcolour in Pink Chocolate.

Yes – much better choice of moisturiser and specialist lifting foundation. The colour choice is also appropriate, but *nothing* has been done to correct the broken veins on the cheeks!

Yes – the eyecolours and blusher match quite nicely, but may emphasise the high colour on the cheeks caused by the broken veins

REJECTED!
Think! This plan can be improved

PLAN C

- Apply a specialist make-up base or primer.
- Moisturiser with SPF8.
- With a soft brush, apply a layer of concealer (green or beige) to the broken veins.
- Treatment foundation in Natural Light Tan applied with a damp cosmetic sponge.
- Light dusting of translucent fine loose powder.
- Highlighter in bone, soft grey eyeshadow, soft black mascara.
- Blusher in Sienne (pinky mauve), small dusting.
- Matt lipcolour in Pink Chocolate.

Yes – a make-up base is a good idea.

Yes – a good choice of moisturiser.

Yes – the concealer would cover the broken veins.

Yes – treatment foundation a good choice, application with a damp sponge will produce a natural finish. Fine loose powder – ok.

Yes – eye and lip colours harmonise, will appear soft and will not clash with high colouring on the cheeks as concealer has been used.

Yes – lip colour matches overall.

CORRECT!

REMEMBER!

When you are answering scenario type questions, you must select a treatment plan which is the most *appropriate* out of the *options given* and not necessarily what *you* would have chosen. Many beauty students train in salons and centres that have fantastic make-up ranges available to them. In fact, some salons update make-up ranges every season!

Examiners ask questions around basic make-up principles only, and not up to the minute products which are outdated the following year. Examiners are not allowed to use proprietary names, nor are they allowed to question candidates about specific cosmetic manufacturers.

Some further scenario examples with correct answers on page 282 are included below.

Scenario One

Q1. Select the most appropriate treatment plan for Mrs Simpson.

A1. Plan selected —————————————

Clients details:
Age 62 years
Retired
Dry, mature skin, lines around eyes and forehead, generally aged, but with good colour and texture
Skin tone pink
Bright grey eyes
Dark eyelashes
Hair tinted (but natural) to mid blonde

Requires:
Natural but special occasion make-up for a wedding

Outfit:
Pink hat
Cream jacket
Pink skirt

PLAN A
- Application of make-up primer base.
- Application of beige tinted moisturiser.
- Application of wand light reflective concealer to naso-labial folds and deeper lines.
- Application of frosted foundation – beige.
- Light dusting of powder.
- White highlighter with Pretty Pink eyeshadow.
- Black mascara.
- Pink blusher.
- Pink lip gloss.

PLAN B
- Application of make-up primer base.
- Application of firming moisturiser.
- Golden tan cream foundation and matching powder.
- Cream highlighter with soft grey eyeshadow.
- Dark grey mascara.
- Mauve blusher to the cheekbones.
- Candy pink lipcolour.
- Shader carefully blended over areas of dropped contours.

PLAN C

- Application of make-up primer base.
- Application of treatment moisturiser.
- Application of wand light reflective concealer on naso-labial folds and deeper lines.
- Natural beige treatment foundation.
- Bone highlighter with soft grey eyeshadow.
- Soft black mascara.
- Blusher in soft mauve.
- Soft mauve matt lipcolour.
- Shader carefully blended over jowl area.

Scenario Two

Q2. Select the most appropriate treatment plan for Miss Mellers.

A2 Plan Selected ————————

Client details:
Age 30 years
Occupation – nurse
Dry, dehydrated skin. Skin colour pale, small pores
Fine appearance, good bone structure
Mid-brown long hair
Very straight eyelashes
Small mouth
Blue eyes
No colour preferences

Requires:
Elegant evening make-up suitable for a formal occasion

Outfit:
Formal black dress

PLAN A

- Application of hydrating moisture lotion.
- Curl eyelashes using eyelash curlers.
- Application of light gold skin illuminator.
- Application of light beige all-in-one powder crème foundation.
- Creamy gold highlighter, golden coffee eyeshadow, dark brown thinly applied eyeliner.
- Dark rich brown mascara.
- Blusher to emphasise eyes and cheekbones in Brown Sand.
- Lip colour in Ginger Frost.
- Application of lip gloss in Clear.
- Spray with mineral water to hydrate and set.

PLAN B

- Application of make-up primer mixed with moisturising cream.
- Application of cream foundation in mid tan.
- Set with translucent powder.
- White highlighter, flannel grey eyeshadow, black, thinly applied eyeliner. Black mascara.
- Blusher to emphasise eyes and cheekbones in mauve.
- Lipcolour in Siren Red matt finish.

PLAN C

- Application of treatment moisturising lotion.
- Application of skin illuminator in beige.
- Application of cream foundation in Pearly Beige Frost.
- Application of frosted loose powder.
- Soft peach highlighter, ginger biscuit eyeshadow, brown highlighter and two layers of black mascara.
- Blusher to emphasise eyes and cheekbones in Blood Orange.
- Application of clear lip gloss to finish.
- Spray with mineral water to hydrate and set.

Scenario Three

Q3. Select the most appropriate treatment plan for Miss Lappin.

A3 Plan selected ——————————

Client details:
Age 24 years
Occupation – secretary
Oily skin
Blemishes around central T Zone area
Open pores
Thick epidermis
Green eyes
Long red hair
Skin colour – even, creamy/ivory

Requires:
Natural, but lasting, bridal make-up

Outfit:
Traditional bridal gown in off-white
Flowers – green and silver foliage with cream roses
Bridesmaids in off-white with emerald green sashes

PLAN A

- Moisturise with liquid moisturiser.
- Apply a pore minimising lotion.
- Apply concealer to the blemished area with a brush.
- Apply a cream foundation all over in Creamy Beige.
- Set with a generous layer of translucent powder pressed well into the T Zone area.
- Ivory highlighter to browbone, Green Aqua eyecolour to the eyelids and two layers of brown mascara.
- Blusher in Pink Haze.
- Lipcolour in Love That Pink.

PLAN B

- Apply an oil absorbing moisturiser.
- Conceal open pores with a pore minimising lotion.
- Apply concealing cream to the blemished T Zone, blend in well.
- Apply a water based foundation in creamy beige.
- Set with translucent powder, press well into the T Zone.
- Apply cream highlighter to the browbone, Soft Lime Green over the eye area and a touch of Moss Green for emphasis.
- Thin layer of dark green eyeliner. Brown mascara.
- Blusher in Tawny Peach, matt lipcolour in Aegean Coral Peach.

PLAN C

- Apply a pre make-up base primer and light moisturiser.
- Apply a layer of powder cream all-in-one foundation in Ivory Beige.
- Ivory highlighter to the browbone with light silver grey to emphasise. Blend the two colours together with a touch of Soft Lime.
- Apply two layers of black lash thickening mascara.
- Blusher in Tawny Peach.
- Lipcolour in Tangerine Gloss.

Answers

SCENARIO ONE – MRS SIMPSON

Correct plan – PLAN C. This plan offered a make-up base, treatment foundation and the corrective make-up available was applied in the correct place, ie:
- to shade the jowls.
- to improve sagging areas around deep lines and the naso-labial folds.

The beige foundation was also a good neutral choice.

The eye colours, blusher and lip colours generally toned in with the outfit and the clients grey eyes.

PLAN A was fundamentally incorrect in offering a frosty foundation and a lip gloss for this mature client.

PLAN B was fundamentally incorrect in offering a Golden Tan foundation, and offering nothing to improve the general loss of contour other than applying shader to the completed make-up.

SCENARIO TWO – MISS MELLERS

Correct plan – PLAN A. This was the only plan to address the problem of the client's 'very straight eyelashes'. The plan also maintained colour harmony throughout. The colours chosen would have suited the client's blue eyes and long brown hair and would have toned with the outfit. The mineral water to hydrate and set was also important for this client.

PLAN B – The foundation choice of mid tan was too dark even for an evening result. The text told us the skin colour was pale. Also the red lipcolour was not really appropriate for a small mouth. Lighter frosty colours would be better accompanied by a lip gloss. Loose powder also can be disastrous for dry, dehydrated skin.

PLAN C started quite well, but a frosty foundation and frosty loose powder was not really appropriate for a dry, dehydrated client of 30 years. The blusher and eyeshadows created a peachy orange theme, but would have been out of balance without the use of a similar toning lipcolour. The lip gloss in neutral was totally inadequate.

SCENARIO THREE – MISS LAPPIN

Correct plan – PLAN B. This was correct because it attempted to meet all the requirements of the bride. The oil-absorbing moisturiser would have minimised shine, and the pore-minimising product would have had the effect of filling in and evening out the open pores. A concealer was also used on blemished areas. The water-based foundation was also appropriate for the oily complexion, duly set with translucent powder. The overall colour choices outlined would have complemented the eye and hair colour and matched the colour theme of the wedding.

PLAN A started off well, but a cream foundation would be inappropriate for such an oily skin, and would soon have resulted in a shiny client. The lipcolour and blusher in pinks could easily have clashed with the client's red hair.

PLAN C did not offer anything to correct or control the oily skin condition, or minimise open pores or blemishes. However, with the exception of the black mascara and the Tangerine Gloss, the colours chosen could have looked quite good. Black mascara would be too harsh for this client, and the lip gloss would probably turn out too shiny on the photographs.

MULTIPLE CHOICE QUESTIONS

Some examples of multiple choice examination questions are included for you to enable you to give yourself a short test. Carefully consider the descriptions provided before choosing your answer. Only one answer is correct.
Indicate your answer by putting an **X** in the circle: ◯

Q1. Sebum is secreted from the:

a) eccrine glands ◯

b) sebaceous glands ◯

c) sweat glands ◯

d) appocrine glands ◯

Q2. The reproducing layer of the epidermis is the stratum:

a) germinitivum ◯

b) lucidum ◯

c) corneum ◯

d) spinosum ◯

Q3. What does overexposure to ultra-violet radiation cause?

a) less melanin to be produced ◯

b) a thicker stratum corneum ◯

c) a reduction in pore size ◯

d) an increase in collagen production ◯

Q4. Which one of the following provide the lower epidermis with food and oxygen?

a) small venules ◯

b) lymph capillaries ◯

c) the dermal papilla ◯

d) small arterioles ◯

Q5. Which statement is correct?

a) the dermis is composed of five scaly layers of cells ◯

b) the dermis is a living structure without nerve endings ◯

c) the dermis lies below the epidermis and above the subcutis ◯

d) the dermis lies below the subcutis ◯

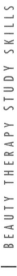

Q6. Which one of the following best describes an oily skin?

a) small pores, shiny appearance ○

b) thin epidermis with broken capillaries ○

c) tight appearance, small pores ○

d) thick epidermis, large pores ○

Q7. What is the best pre make-up base for an oily complexion?

a) an oil-absorbing moisturiser ○

b) a moisturising cream ○

c) a spray of mineral water ○

d) a moisturiser containing a humectant ○

Q8. What is a suitable foundation product for a dry, lined skin?

a) a medicated foundation ○

b) a cream foundation ○

c) a liquid foundation ○

d) a mousse-type foundation ○

Q9. If a client required a heavy coverage from the foundation application, which one of the following would *not* be recommended?

a) a powder cream foundation ○

b) a cream foundation ○

c) an all-in-one foundation ○

d) a liquid foundation ○

Q10. A client with a florid skin tone should be advised to use

a) a tinted moisturiser in a Tan shade ○

b) a medium coverage rose beige foundation ○

c) a thicker coverage flat beige foundation ○

d) a mauve tinted corrective colour wash ○

Q11. What is a common ingredient in lipstick?

a) petroleum jelly ○

b) chalk ○

c) paraffin wax ○

d) calcium thioglycollate ○

Q12. Which one of the following is used to produce a frosting effect in eyeshadows and lip cosmetics?

a) waxes ○

b) mica ○

c) silicone ○

d) paraben ○

Q13. Conjunctivitis is a bacterial infection which affects the:

a) nose and mouth ○

b) scalp ○

c) eyes ○

d) skin ○

Q14. Which one of the following is caused by a virus?

a) impetigo ○

b) psoriasis ○

c) tinea circinata ○

d) herpes simplex ○

Q15. If the therapist suspects the client has a contagious condition, the correct course of action is to:

a) carry out the make-up treatment and sterilise all brushes and palettes afterwards ○

b) tactfully advise the client to visit their GP ○

c) continue with the make-up treatment and omit the suspect area ○

d) discuss the client's condition with a senior colleague ○

Q16. The best way to clean and disinfect make-up brushes is to:

a) wash them in hot soapy water and then in a disinfectant solution; dry naturally ○

b) wipe the brushes over with a 70% alcohol substance; dry naturally ○

c) place the brushes in a UV cabinet for 30 minutes; turn the brushes regularly ○

d) wash them in a hot antiseptic solution and allow them to dry naturally ○

Q17. As part of the disinfection process, make-up trays should be wiped over with:

a) an antiseptic ○

b) a hypochlorite ○

c) a 20% alcohol solution ○

d) rosewater ○

Q18. Full and complete make-up records should be available for each client because:

a) the client pays for this service in the price of the make-up treatment ○

b) it helps with the reordering of stock ○

c) it provides a reference that enables the therapist to recreate that particular make-up ○

d) it is general salon policy ○

Q19. Which one of the following is considered to be the perfect face shape?

a) heart ○

b) round ○

c) square ○

d) oval ○

Q20. The best way to improve the appearance of a crooked nose is to:

a) apply shader to areas that need straightening ○

b) apply highlighter to the centre of the nose ○

c) apply highlighter to the areas that need straightening ○

d) apply shader to the sides of the nose ○

Q21. A small, undersized mouth can be made to look fuller by the use of:

a) lip pencil that outlines the natural shape ○

b) strong, deep matt colours ○

c) pale, pearly lip colours ○

d) lip balm ○

The following three questions refer to the text below:

> Holly has a dry, sensitive skin type. Brown eyes and hair. She requires a natural daytime make-up.

Q22. What products should be used to cleanse and tone the skin prior to the make-up application?

a) a cream cleanser and orangeflower water ○

b) hypoallergenic cleansing emulsion and rosewater ○

c) a wash off cleanser and witch hazel ○

d) a cleansing lotion and orangeflower water ○

Q23. The client has selected a Bronze eyeshadow theme and a Brown Coffee Bean lip colour. Which of the following mascara colours best complement the overall theme?

a) grey ○

b) soft black ○

c) navy ○

d) brown ○

Q24. Which one of the following products will moisturise the
skin and impart a very natural effect?

a) a tinted moisturiser   ◯

b) a bronzing powder   ◯

c) a foundation cream   ◯

d) an all-in-one foundation   ◯

Q25. A standard filament lamp is not considered as suitable
lighting for make-up application because:

a) it is too bright for the client's eyes   ◯

b) it makes red tones appear darker   ◯

c) it makes red and blue tones appear less intense   ◯

d) it makes the make-up application appear unnatural   ◯

MULTIPLE CHOICE TEST – ANSWERS

1.	B	6.	D	11.	A	16.	A	21.	C
2.	A	7.	A	12.	B	17.	B	22.	B
3.	B	8.	B	13.	C	18.	C	23.	D
4.	D	9.	D	14.	D	19.	D	24.	A
5.	C	10.	C	15.	B	20.	A	25.	B

Marking and Grading

All correct   excellent, well done

20 correct   very well done

15 correct   ok, but go back to your notes and Revision Maps and see
if you can improve your score

Less than 10   You need to go back and spend some time revising

FINAL END TEST

This section consists of statements. Each one may be correct or incorrect. The answer required is simply

Yes or No.

In your assessment of whether the statement is correct or incorrect, you must only base your answer on the information provided. The questions are arranged in groups in the order that the related topics occurred in the text. After ensuring that all the questions have been answered, check the answers yourself in the back of the book.

• FINAL END TEST

1. An area of severe bruising is a contra-indication to make-up application.

2. A client who is extremely sensitive should undergo a make-up treatment using hypoallergenic products.

3. A severe acne condition is a contra-indication to make-up application because it could be worsened or inflamed.

4. It is not important that the client agrees the make-up plan.

5. Details of the bridesmaids' outfits and flowers should be ascertained during a bridal make-up consultation.

6. An evening make-up application requires a lighter textured foundation to be used.

7. Frosted foundations should be avoided if the skin is lined or crepey.

8. Pre make-up bases can add to the lasting properties of the make-up.

9. Corrective colour washes should be used on all skin types.

10. Gel foundations are suitable for tanned or black clients.

11. Cream foundation is suitable for all skin types.

12. Blushers are used to enhance the eyes and give vitality to the face.

13. Loose powder contains magnesium carbonate for absorption.

14. Pressed powder is suitable for touching up a make-up, but not for setting a foundation application.

15. Mascara and eye cosmetics can be best removed using an eye make-up remover.

16. A common ingredient in mascara is silk particles.

17. Eyeshadows contain talc, oils and pigments.

18. Eyeshadows contain the strongest colour pigments.

19. Highlighters are used to bring forward or emphasise areas of the face.

20. A lip pencil is harder than a lipstick.

21. A lipstick contains an oil (like castor oil) to soften and lubricate the lips.

22. There is no advantage to the use of cosmetics with a SPF (Sun Protection Factor).

23. A square face can be softened by the use of highlighter on the jawbone.

24. A pear face shape can be improved by highlighting the sides of the forehead and shading the widest part of the jawline.

25. Sharpening an eye pencil prior to use can reduce the presence of micro-organisms.

26. Lip gloss is recommended for a person with a small mouth.

27. A double chin or jowls can be diminished by applying shader or a darker foundation to the relaxed area.

28. Mirrors and make-up trays can be wiped over with a 70% alcohol solution as part of the sanitisation process.

29. Clients who wear glasses with heavy frames will require more muted lip colours.

30. If the eyes are wide apart, use lighter colours to the outer edges and darker colours to the inner eyelid.

31. A suitable choice of mascara for a client with white hair is a soft grey.

32. Cover sticks conceal minor blemishes, but are not suitable for concealing large areas of pigmentation.

33. Make-up sponges should be washed out and soaked in a hypochlorite solution after use to maintain optimum hygiene.

34. Generally, wine-coloured blushers are more effective on black skins than peaches and pinks.

35. Transparent gel foundations are ideal on darker complexions, especially if the skin is blemish-free.

FINAL END TEST **ANSWERS**

1. Yes
2. Yes
3. Yes
4. No   Quite untrue. The client should be fully involved in devising the make-up plan, and client should *sign* the make-up plan.
5. Yes
6. No   A thicker foundation offering a more complete coverage is more appropriate for an evening make-up application.
7. Yes
8. Yes
9. No   Use only if the skin colour is sallow or florid.
10. Yes
11. No   Not correct. Cream foundation is more suitable for a dry, mature skin.
12. Yes
13. Yes
14. Yes
15. Yes
16. Yes
17. Yes
18. No   Blusher actually has the strongest pigments.
19. Yes
20. Yes
21. Yes
22. No   This is not true. Any products with an SPF will protect the face from the damaging effect of UV rays.
23. No   Shader, not highlighter, should be used on the corners of the jawbone.
24. Yes
25. Yes
26. Yes
27. Yes

28. Yes   Remember, anything below 70% alcohol is not classed as a disinfectant.

29. No   Stronger frames mean the lip colour and the eye colours will need to be bolder to give balance.

30. Yes

31. Yes

32. Yes   A camouflage-type cream or a concealing cream would be better as these products have more pigment and would cover more effectively.

33. Yes

34. Yes

35. Yes

Marking and Grading

The marking guide is provided to help and encourage you to monitor your progress. This style of end test has been chosen to reinforce some key revision points to further assist your revision process. Obviously, if you have guessed a lot of the answers, it will not give you a proper reflection of the true mark you have achieved, and really, if you have needed to guess answers, you need to revise a bit more.

28 correct answers   a credit

25 correct answers   a confident pass

21 correct answers   a borderline pass

Below 21 correct means you need to revise a bit more. Go back to your course notes and Revision Maps, spend some more time studying, and have another go at the test at a later date. Don't be put off, but be prepared to spend some proper time on it.

CHECKLIST ✓ Can You?

		Yes	No	Page No
1.	Recognise some basic hair terminology.			297
2.	Explain the position of the hair within the structure of the skin (Chapter 3).			106
3.	Explain the stages of the hair growth cycle: anagen, catagen, telogen.			298
4.	Discuss alternative methods of temporary hair removal.			299
5.	List the possible causes of excessive hair growth in women.			300
6.	Write accurately about the features of different waxing methods, and the lightening of superfluous hair.			301
7.	State general and specific contra-indications to waxing and sugaring treatments.			305
8.	List safety precautions that must be observed during waxing and sugaring treatments.			306
9.	State contra-indications and safety precautions relevant to bleaching or lightening of superfluous hair.			307
10.	Complete a final end test.			317

WAXING AND LIGHTENING HAIR

In order to carry out these beauty treatments, you need to understand the hair growth cycle.

Also, revisit the Revision Map around skin structure: you should be sure about the position of the hair in the skin (Chapter 3).

Review your course notes so that your knowledge of hygiene, contra-indications, safety precautions and providing treatments is first rate.

Revision Maps have been provided around some popular examination question areas. A Revision Map is provided around the possible causes of superfluous hair growth, but this knowledge is not a requirement for every awarding body.

Some short answer questions are provided for you, and a complete multiple choice examination paper and end test complete the chapter.

SHORT ANSWER QUESTIONS

An example of some model questions and answers are provided to help give you an insight on how to answer questions properly. Reading through the questions and answers will also help your revision.

Q1. Outline the hair growth cycle. *(10 marks)*

Answer: The hair growth cycle is quite simply a process of growth, change, rest and repeat.

The growing stage is termed the Anagen stage. Rapid activity takes place in the hair follicle as it rebuilds itself growing downwards, ready to accommodate a new hair. The papilla cells and hair germ cells start to grow. Many cell changes take place, until finally the hair as we know it emerges at the top of the follicle. The hair is now a fully formed anagen hair, comfortably settled in the hair follicle and nourished by the dermal papilla. The hair can remain in anagen for a period of weeks or years.

When the nourishment from the dermal papilla stops, the hair breaks away from the follicle base; the root-like base of the hair disappears and is replaced by a brush-like base. This is called a club hair. The follicle base begins to shrink. This is a time of change, or the *catagen* stage.

Revision Map – Some Key Hair Terminology

Some Hair Terminology

The Hair
- Dead keratinous structure.
- Grows out of the follicle at an angle to the skin.
- Follows body contours.
- Follows a growth cycle.

Anagen → Catagen → Telogen

or

Growth → Change → Rest → Repeat

Hair Follicle
Sac or pocket which holds the hair.

Vellus Hair
- Downy.
- Soft body/facial hair.

Terminal Hair
- Coarser.
- Stronger.
- Deeper roots.
- Some are for protection, eg eyebrows.

Dermal Papilla
- Where active cells start to grow.
- Has a good blood supply.

Sebaceous Gland
- Situated in dermis.
- Opens into hair follicle.
- Sebum lubricates hair and skin.

Hair Shaft
Part of the hair visible above the skin.

Hair Root
Part of the hair below skin's surface, towards the base of follicle.

Superfluous Hair
Is unwanted, but not abnormal, hair growth.

Hypertrichosis
Abnormal excessive hair growth.

Revision Map – The Stages of Hair Growth

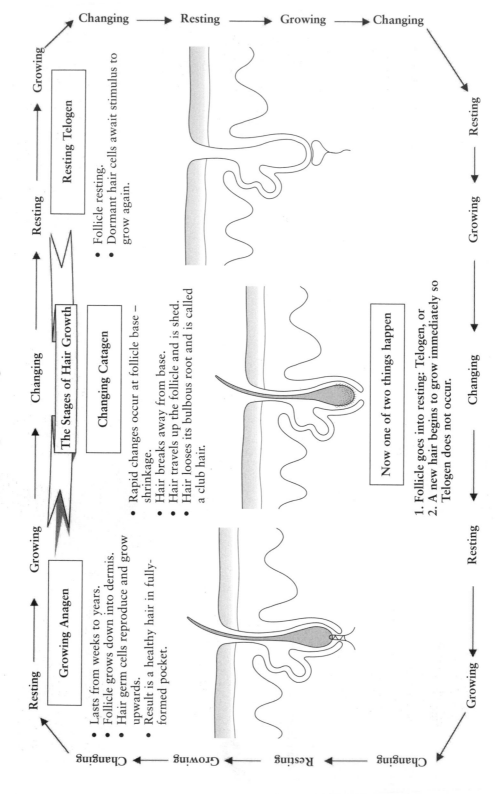

Changing → Resting → Growing → Changing

Growing Anagen

- Lasts from weeks to years.
- Follicle grows down into dermis.
- Hair germ cells reproduce and grow upwards.
- Result is a healthy hair in fully-formed pocket.

The Stages of Hair Growth

Changing Catagen

- Rapid changes occur at follicle base – shrinkage.
- Hair breaks away from base.
- Hair travels up the follicle and is shed.
- Hair looses its bulbous root and is called a club hair.

Resting Telogen

- Follicle resting.
- Dormant hair cells await stimulus to grow again.

Now one of two things happen

1. Follicle goes into resting: Telogen, or
2. A new hair begins to grow immediately so Telogen does not occur.

Resting → Growing → Changing → Resting

Growing

Changing

Resting

Growing

Changing

Revision Map – Alternative Methods of Temporary Hair Removal

Alternative Temporary Methods of Hair Removal

Shaving
- Cuts hair at skin's surface so it is bristly when it grows through.
- Inexpensive.
- Modern razors and shaving products have improved this method.

Threading
- Popular with Asian clientele.
- Cotton thread is carefully worked to remove excess hair.
- Same effect as plucking.

Plucking
- OK for eyebrows.
- Hairs can grow back thicker.

Abrasive Mitts
- Rubbed over the area in a circular motion.
- Used on legs.
- Inexpensive.
- Exfoliating so skin feels smooth after use.

Cutting
- Scissors.
- OK for moles or trimming between electrolysis.
- Leaves a bristly surface.

Cold Wax Strips
- Cellophane strips coated with cold wax.
- Not very effective.
- Not many clients can remove strips quickly.
- Expensive.

Epil Shaving
- Electric shaving system.
- Has effect of mass plucking.
- Painful.
- Expensive to purchase initially.

Depilatory Creams
- Procuct is keratolytic; it dissolves keratin.
- Removes hair by chemical action just below skin's surface. Common ingredient is calcium thioglycollate.
- Car. cause allergic reaction.
- Can sensitise skin if used a lot.
- Smells awful.
- Quite expensive.

Revision Map – Possible Causes of Excessive Hair Growth in Women

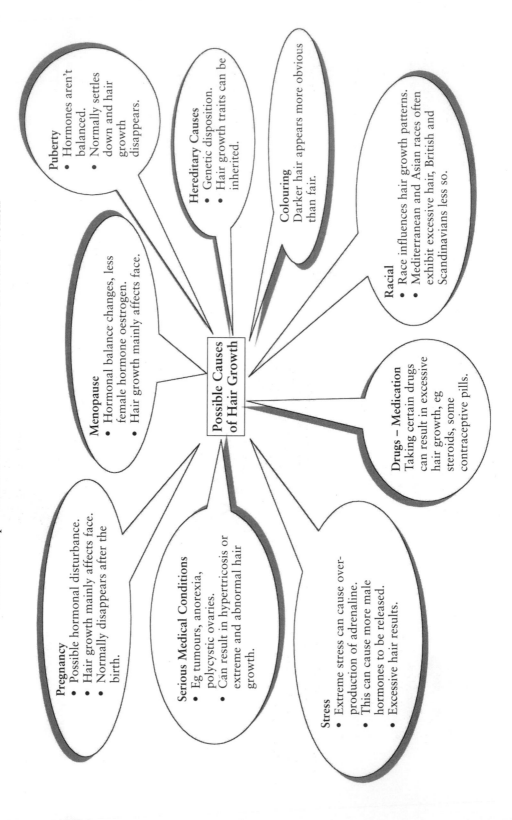

Possible Causes of Hair Growth

Puberty
- Hormones aren't balanced.
- Normally settles down and hair growth disappears.

Hereditary Causes
- Genetic disposition.
- Hair growth traits can be inherited.

Colouring
Darker hair appears more obvious than fair.

Racial
- Race influences hair growth patterns.
- Mediterranean and Asian races often exhibit excessive hair, British and Scandinavians less so.

Menopause
- Hormonal balance changes, less female hormone oestrogen.
- Hair growth mainly affects face.

Drugs – Medication
Taking certain drugs can result in excessive hair growth, eg steroids, some contraceptive pills.

Pregnancy
- Possible hormonal disturbance.
- Hair growth mainly affects face.
- Normally disappears after the birth.

Serious Medical Conditions
- Eg tumours, anorexia, polycystic ovaries.
- Can result in hypertricosis or extreme and abnormal hair growth.

Stress
- Extreme stress can cause over-production of adrenaline.
- This can cause more male hormones to be released.
- Excessive hair results.

Revision Map – Features of Warm wax

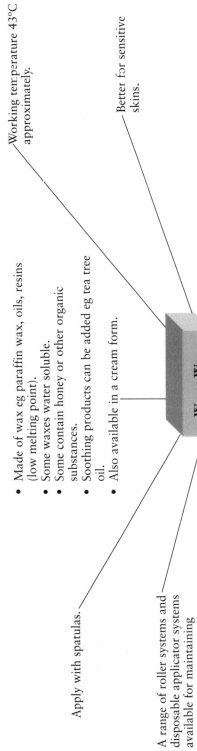
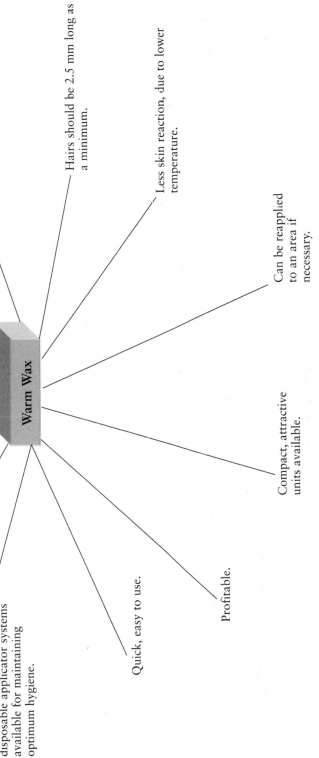

Warm Wax

- Made of wax eg paraffin wax, oils, resins (low melting point).
- Some waxes water soluble.
- Some contain honey or other organic substances.
- Soothing products can be added eg tea tree oil.
- Also available in a cream form.

Working temperature 43°C approximately.

Better for sensitive skins.

Hairs should be 2.5 mm long as a minimum.

Less skin reaction, due to lower temperature.

Can be reapplied to an area if necessary.

Compact, attractive units available.

Profitable.

Quick, easy to use.

A range of roller systems and disposable applicator systems available for maintaining optimum hygiene.

Apply with spatulas.

Revision Map – Features of Hot Wax

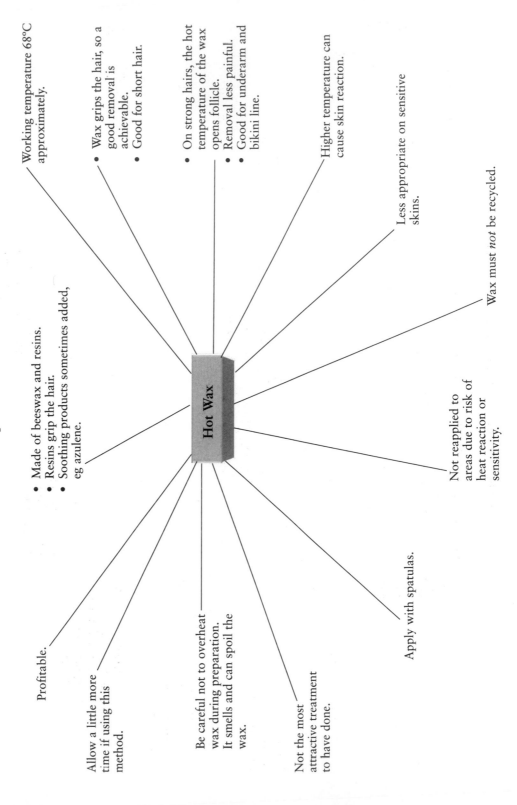

Hot Wax

- Made of beeswax and resins.
- Resins grip the hair.
- Soothing products sometimes added, eg azulene.

Working temperature 68°C approximately.

- Wax grips the hair, so a good removal is achievable.
- Good for short hair.

- On strong hairs, the hot temperature of the wax opens follicle.
- Removal less painful.
- Good for underarm and bikini line.

Higher temperature can cause skin reaction.

Less appropriate on sensitive skins.

Wax must *not* be recycled.

Not reapplied to areas due to risk of heat reaction or sensitivity.

Apply with spatulas.

Not the most attractive treatment to have done.

Be careful not to overheat wax during preparation. It smells and can spoil the wax.

Allow a little more time if using this method.

Profitable.

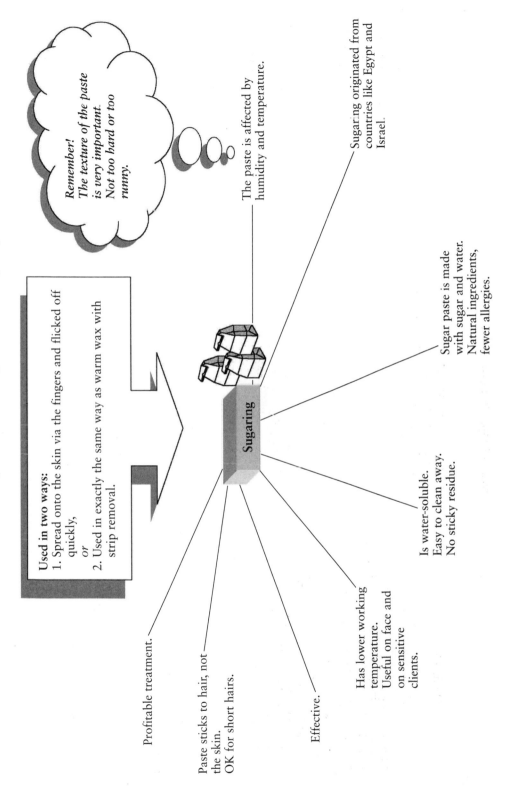

Revision Map – Features of Sugar Paste and Sugaring

Used in two ways:
1. Spread onto the skin *via* the fingers and flicked off quickly,
or
2. Used in exactly the same way as warm wax with strip removal.

Remember!
The texture of the paste is very important.
Not too hard or too runny.

The paste is affected by humidity and temperature.

Sugaring originated from countries like Egypt and Israel.

Sugar paste is made with sugar and water. Natural ingredients, fewer allergies.

Sugaring

Is water-soluble. Easy to clean away. No sticky residue.

Has lower working temperature. Useful on face and on sensitive clients.

Effective.

Paste sticks to hair, not the skin. OK for short hairs.

Profitable treatment.

Revision Map – Features of Bleaching Excessive Hair, and how Bleaching works

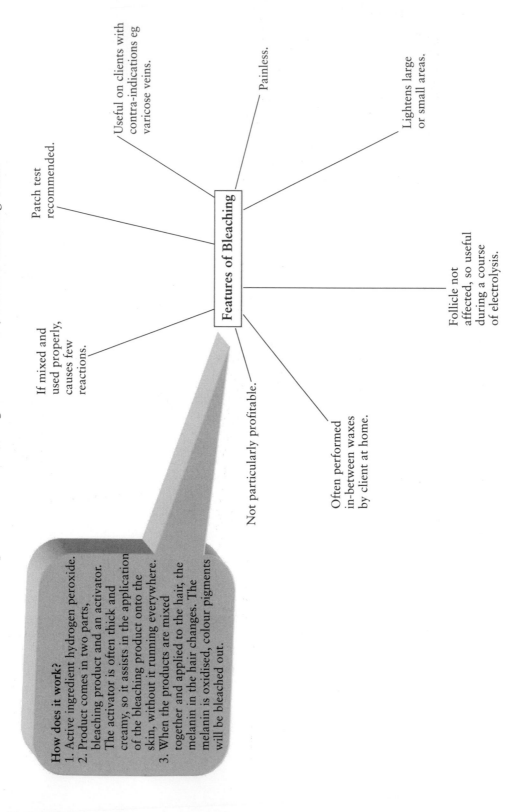

Features of Bleaching

Patch test recommended.

Useful on clients with contra-indications eg varicose veins.

Painless.

Lightens large or small areas.

Follicle not affected, so useful during a course of electrolysis.

Often performed in-between waxes by client at home.

Not particularly profitable.

If mixed and used properly, causes few reactions.

How does it work?
1. Active ingredient hydrogen peroxide.
2. Product comes in two parts, bleaching product and an activator. The activator is often thick and creamy, so it assists in the application of the bleaching product onto the skin, without it running everywhere.
3. When the products are mixed together and applied to the hair, the melanin in the hair changes. The melanin is oxidised, colour pigments will be bleached out.

Revision Map – Contra-indications to Waxing and Sugaring

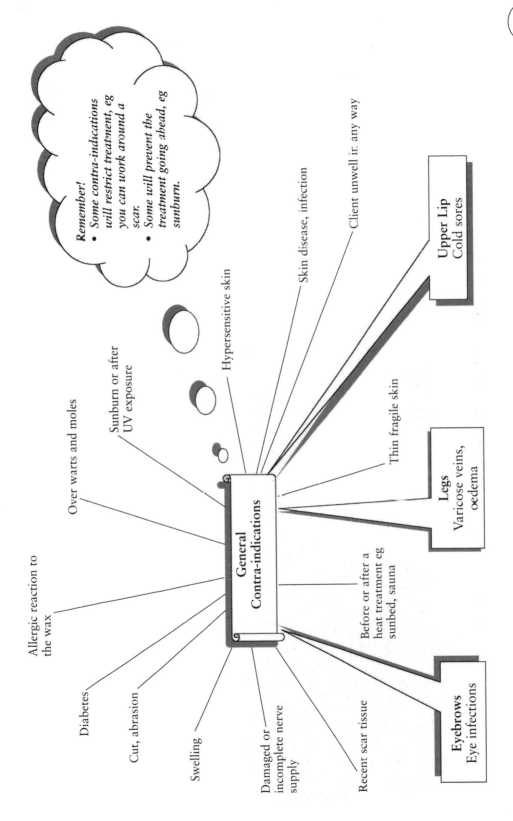

Remember!
- Some contra-indications will restrict treatment, eg you can work around a scar:
- Some will prevent the treatment going ahead, eg sunburn.

Allergic reaction to the wax

Over warts and moles

Sunburn or after UV exposure

Hypersensitive skin

Skin disease, infection

Client unwell ir any way

Diabetes

Cut, abrasion

Swelling

Damaged or incomplete nerve supply

Recent scar tissue

Before or after a heat treatment eg sunbed, sauna

Thin fragile skin

General Contra-indications

Upper Lip
Cold sores

Legs
Varicose veins, oedema

Eyebrows
Eye infections

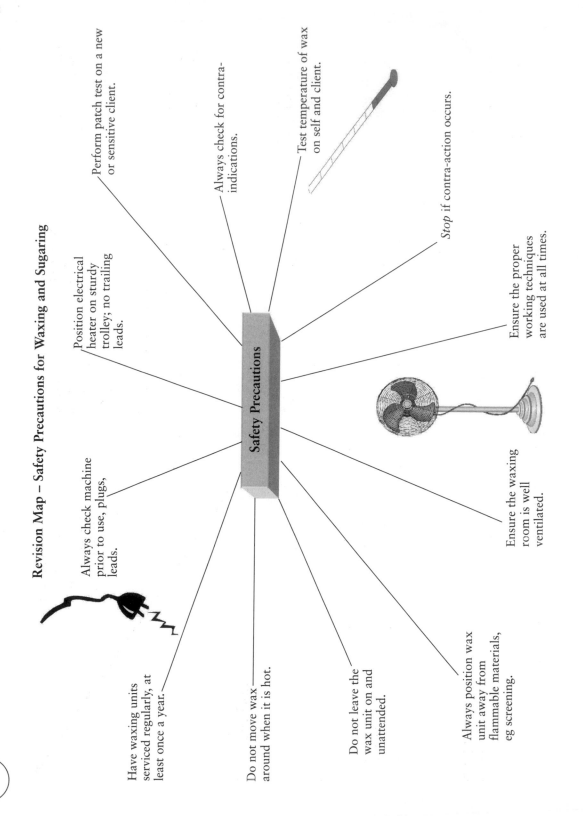

Revision Map – Safety Precautions for Waxing and Sugaring

Safety Precautions

Perform patch test on a new or sensitive client.

Always check for contra-indications.

Test temperature of wax on self and client.

Stop if contra-action occurs.

Position electrical heater on sturdy trolley; no trailing leads.

Ensure the proper working techniques are used at all times.

Always check machine prior to use, plugs, leads.

Ensure the waxing room is well ventilated.

Have waxing units serviced regularly, at least once a year.

Do not move wax around when it is hot.

Do not leave the wax unit on and unattended.

Always position wax unit away from flammable materials, eg screening.

Revision Map – Contra-indications and Safety Precautions for Bleaching of Excess Hair

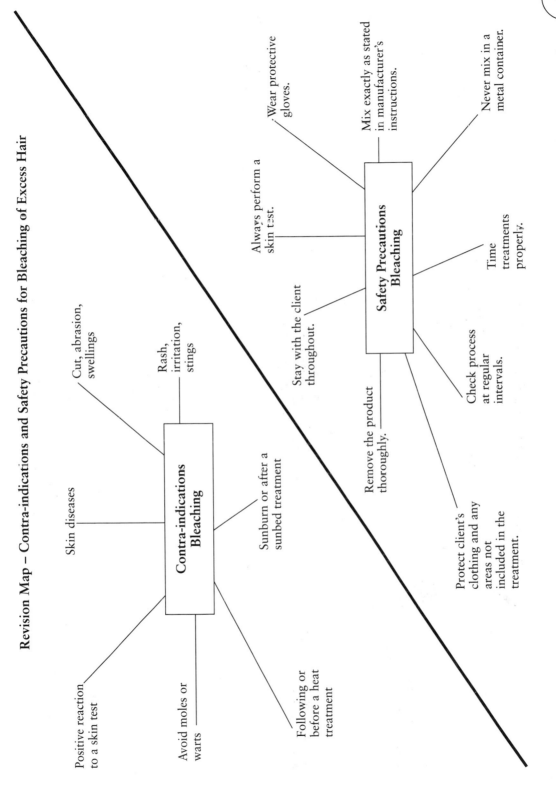

Contra-indications Bleaching

- Cut, abrasion, swellings
- Rash, irritation, stings
- Skin diseases
- Positive reaction to a skin test
- Avoid moles or warts
- Following or before a heat treatment
- Sunburn or after a sunbed treatment

Safety Precautions Bleaching

- Wear protective gloves.
- Mix exactly as stated in manufacturer's instructions.
- Never mix in a metal container.
- Always perform a skin test.
- Stay with the client throughout.
- Time treatments properly.
- Check process at regular intervals.
- Remove the product thoroughly.
- Protect client's clothing and any areas not included in the treatment.

Following the Catagen stage, the hair is shed and the follicle will either go into a rest or Telogen stage, or it may start to grow a new hair immediately.

In a true Telogen stage, the follicle shrinks. This time of rest does not last long, normally 2–3 weeks. More often than not, in the healthy individual a new growth cycle is started immediately.

Q2. What is the method for hot depilatory wax application? *(2 marks)*

Answer: The initial stroke is always against the hair growth, usually followed by a stroke with the hair growth, and a final one against. The idea is to build up a pliable layer so removal is achieved without breaking the hair. Spatulas are always used.

Q3. How should surgical spirit be stored? Why? *(3 marks)*

Answer: In a cool, dry place in the original sealed container. A metal cupboard is the ideal place to store surgical spirit. This product comes under COSHH regulations, is highly inflammable and should not be inhaled.

Q4. In what circumstances should patch testing be carried out prior to a waxing treatment? *(2 marks)*

Answer:
- If the client has a history of allergic reaction to cosmetic products.
- If the skin appeared fine or sensitive.
- If it was the first waxing treatment for the client.

Q5. Define simply the term telogen. *(1 mark)*

Answer: This refers to the resting stage of the hair growth cycle.

Q6. What is the working temperature of hot depilatory wax? *(1 mark)*

Answer: 68°C approximately.

Q7. In depilatory waxing, what factors influence the choice of product and procedure for the client? Justify your answer. *(8 marks)*

Answer:

• The condition of the client's skin is a very important consideration. A drier, more sensitive skin would be more suitable for waxing with warm wax or sugar paste, rather than hot wax, which requires a higher working temperature.

• The area to be treated is also important. Whereas hot wax is excellent for underarm and bikini line it is less popular for facial waxing and leg waxing.

• The density and coarseness of the hair must also be considered. A strong hair growth over a larger area may be more suitable for the use of hot wax, or even a roll-on warm wax system which heats the wax to a higher temperature.

• The preferences of the client should also be considered. The natural aspect of a sugar paste treatment may appeal to one client, but would not be the preference of another.

• The time available is also an important consideration. Warm waxing is an extremely quick, manageable treatment, so might be chosen if the client was trying to fit in a waxing treatment during a lunch break.

Q8. State four advantages of regular waxing or sugaring treatments. *(4 marks)*

Answer:
• The results are instant: the area is cleared of excess hair.
• The results can last 6–8 weeks depending on the individual.
• Re-growth hair appears finer, and over time it is not unusual for sparser hair growth to appear.
• The treatment is quick, should not be painful, and is relatively inexpensive.

Q9. Give two disadvantages of depilatory waxing. *(2 marks)*

Answer:
• If proper home care is not adhered to, ingrowing hairs can occur.
• In very few clients, skin reactions can occur. These often subside after 48 hours but can be very unpleasant at the time.
• For clients who need a lot of areas waxed regularly the cost can be prohibitive.

Q10. Why is talcum powder applied to the area to be waxed? *(1 mark)*

Answer: To ensure that the area is dry, and to raise the hairs from the skin's surface.

Q11. a) Why are diabetic clients contra-indicated to treatment?
b) Are there any occasions when diabetic clients can have a waxing treatment? If so, which wax could be used? *(6 marks)*

Answer: a) Diabetic clients have a lowered resistance to infection, and heal more slowly. Their circulation is also sometimes impaired and they have a reduced sensitivity to heat. Thus their reaction to a waxing treatment is unpredictable.
b) Clients with written GP approval can undergo a waxing treatment (providing they have no other contra-indications). Hot wax should never be used. Warm waxing systems would be recommended or strip sugaring, due to their lower working temperatures. Ideally, the use of a disposable applicator system should be employed, as they are most hygienic.

Q12. What should be applied to the skin following a waxing treatment?
(1 mark)

Answer: A soothing after-wax product, eg after-wax lotion.

Q13. How should the legs be prepared for a waxing treatment? *(4 marks)*

Answer:
• Careful examination of the area for contra-indications.
• Careful examination of the skin and hair growth.
• Wiping over with an antiseptic pre-waxing product.
• Drying the area.
• Applying a light dusting of talc to ensure the area is dry and to lift the hair from the skin's surface.
• Covering any moles, scars or tags with petroleum jelly.

Q14. State one contra-indication specific to eyebrow waxing. *(1 mark)*

Answer: Conjunctivitis (or stye, swelling, or during a hay fever attack).

Q15. How is hot wax recycled? *(1 mark)*

Answer: Hot wax is *never* reused or recycled in any way.

Q16. Why does an area often appear red and spotty after treatment? *(2 marks)*

Answer: This is a normal reaction caused by the extra blood that arrives at the follicles as a result of the waxing treatment. This normally disappears within 24 hours of the treatment.

Q17. What is vellus hair? *(1 mark)*

Answer: This is soft downy hair, often found on the body.

Q18. What is a terminal hair? *(2 marks)*

Answer: These are hairs which are longer and coarser than vellus hair. They can have a protective role, eg eyebrows/lashes.

Q19. How does a depilatory cream work? *(2 marks)*

Answer: A depilatory cream contains a chemical, eg calcium thioglycollate, that dissolves the hair just below the skin's surface.

Q20. What is meant by the term 'the hair in catagen'? *(5 marks)*

Answer: This refers to the time of change in the hair growth cycle when the hair breaks away from the follicle base. The hair loses its bulbous root and its base takes on a fragmented appearance. The hair is eventually shed. As this occurs, the base of the follicle also experiences rapid changes – it degenerates and shrinks.

Q21. Name the gland that lubricates the skin and hair. *(1 mark)*

Answer: The sebaceous gland.

Q22. In the hair growth cycle, what does the term an anagen hair mean?
(2 marks)
Give two features of an anagen hair. *(2 marks)*

Answer: An anagen hair is a growing hair in the follicle. It has a rich blood supply via the dermal papilla, and is situated comfortably in the hair follicle.

In anagen, the follicle is approximately six times longer than in a telogen condition. The anagen stage can last from weeks to years, but ceases when the hair becomes detached from the dermal papilla.

Q23. State five safety precautions applicable to waxing treatments. *(5 marks)*

Answer:
• Always check the machine prior to use, eg plugs, leads.
• Position electrical equipment on a sturdy trolley and ensure that there are no trailing leads.
• Perform a patch test on a new or sensitive client.
• Always check the client for contra-indications.
• Always test temperature of wax on yourself and the client.
• Stop immediately if a contra-action occurs.
• Ensure the proper working techniques are used at all times.
• Have waxing units checked and serviced regularly.
• Do not move the wax unit around whilst hot.
• Do not leave the wax unit on and unattended.
• Always position the unit away from flammable materials eg screening.
• Ensure the waxing room is well ventilated.

MULTIPLE CHOICE QUESTIONS

Some examples of multiple choice examination questions are included for you to enable you to give yourself a short test. Carefully consider the descriptions provided before choosing your answer. Only one answer is correct.
Indicate your answer by putting an **X** in the circle: ◯

Q1. Which regulations state that wax heaters must be serviced regularly?
a) COSHH 1988 ◯
b) Electricity at Work 1990 ◯
c) Employer's Liability Insurance 1969 ◯
d) The Code of Ethics ◯

Q2. Which one of the following could *restrict* an underarm waxing treatment?
a) mastitis ◯
b) overlong hair growth ◯
c) a mole ◯
d) swollen lymph nodes ◯

Q3. How should the eyebrow area be prepared prior to waxing?

a) remove eye make-up and wipe over with a mild antiseptic pre-waxing product ○

b) remove eye make-up with hypoallergenic eye make-up remover ○

c) wipe over the area with rosewater ○

d) remove eye make-up and apply a hot compress to open the pores ○

Q4. Sugaring is especially useful for providing facial waxing treatment because:

a) it is more profitable for the salon ○

b) its working temperature is higher, so a good root lift is possible ○

c) it grips coarser hair, leaving natural downy hair behind ○

d) it can be recycled ○

Q5. Gloves are worn during waxing treatments because:

a) they look clinical ○

b) they act as a protective barrier between the client and the operator ○

c) they are costed into the treatment price ○

d) they protect the operator from burning their hands ○

Q6. The most common ingredients of hot wax are:

a) sugar water and resins ○

b) organic honey and resins ○

c) beeswax and resins ○

d) paraffin wax and resins ○

Q7. Hot wax is often the treatment choice for strong underarm hair because:

a) its working temperature is higher, so it opens the follicle, ensuring a less painful and clean removal ○

b) it is more hygienic as it is disposable ○

c) it can be applied in small sections if the hair growth is irregular ○

d) it is water-soluble, so any residue can be removed without irritation ○

Q8. The hair is nourished in the follicle via the:

a) arrector pili ○

b) sebaceous gland ○

c) dermis ○

d) dermal papilla ○

Q9. In the hair growth cycle the term catagen refers to a time of:

a) regrowth ○

b) change ○

c) growth ○

d) rest ○

Q10. The active ingredient in depilatory creams is:

a) azulene ○

b) hydrogen peroxide ○

c) ammonia ○

d) calcium thioglycollate ○

Q11. Clients with a sensitive skin type are generally more suitable for hair removal by:

a) hot waxing ○

b) warm waxing ○

c) sugaring ○

d) bleaching ○

Q12. Appropriate leg waxing aftercare advice for a client prone to ingrowing hairs would be:

a) exfoliate weekly, use shower gel when showering ○

b) exfoliate daily using exfoliating granules ○

c) exfoliate and apply body lotion three times a week ○

d) exfoliate gently and apply moisturiser daily ○

Q13. The active ingredient in bleaching products is:

a) hydrogen peroxide

b) accelerator

c) potassium hydroxide

d) formaldehyde

Q14. Processing time for lightening thick *dark brown* hair is most likely to be:

a) 2–5 minutes

b) 5–10 minutes

c) 10–15 minutes

d) 20–25 minutes

Q15. Bleaching products should *not* be mixed in a:

a) metal dish

b) plastic dish

c) ceramic dish

d) glass dish

Q16. Which of the following is a contra-indication to bleaching?

a) following a sunbed treatment

b) nervous clients

c) a negative reaction to a skin test

d) the client is allergic to depilatory creams

Q17. The working temperature of warm wax is approximately:

a) 34°C

b) 43°C

c) 55°C

d) 68°C

Q18. Applying warm wax too thickly could result in:

a) a skin reaction

b) better hair removal

c) a less painful treatment

d) less effective hair removal

Q19. Terminal hair is:

a) downy and soft ○

b) strong and coarse ○

c) found only on the scalp ○

d) shed after birth ○

Q20. Perfumed body lotion should not be applied following waxing as:

a) the follicle is open and irritation could occur ○

b) the client may dislike the fragrance ○

c) the product is more expensive than after-wax lotion ○

d) the product does not contain anything antiseptic ○

MULTIPLE CHOICE TEST – ANSWERS

1.	B	6.	C	11.	C	16.	A
2.	C	7.	A	12.	D	17.	B
3.	A	8.	D	13.	A	18.	D
4.	C	9.	B	14.	C	19.	B
5.	B	10.	D	15.	A	20.	A

Marking and Grading

16 correct   a credit, excellent

12 correct   a pass, well done

Just below 10   you're nearly there. Keep revising, review the Revision Maps and have another go

Below 5   you need to spend more time revising. Look again at your course notes and the Revision Maps, and have another go in a week's time

FINAL END TEST

This section consists of statements. Each one may be correct or incorrect. The answer required is simply

Yes or No.

In your assessment of whether the statement is correct or incorrect, you must only base your answer on the information provided. The questions are arranged in groups in the order that the related topics occurred in the text. After ensuring that all the questions have been answered, check the answers yourself at the end of the chapter.

• FINAL END TEST

1. Conjunctivitis would *not* contra-indicate an eyebrow waxing or sugaring treatment.

2. If a client had a severe varicose condition, they could be recommended to have a bleaching treatment.

3. Moles and skin tags can be coated with petroleum jelly and avoided during underarm waxing.

4. Thicker hair growth in the bikini line can be removed less painfully with hot wax.

5. The working temperature of hot wax is approximately 68°C.

6. The ingredients of hot wax are commonly beeswax and resins.

7. In hot waxing the resin grips the hair.

8. Hot wax is more suitable for sensitive skin.

9. Sugar paste can be used with strips, the effect is the same as warm waxing.

10. Sugar paste contains only natural ingredients.

11. Sugar paste is *not* water-soluble.

12. Warm wax takes 20–30 minutes to heat up thoroughly.

13. Warm wax is applied *thinly* in the same direction as the hair growth.

14. Common ingredients in warm wax are paraffin wax or honey.

15. In warm wax the hairs are coated with the wax. They are depilated when the strip is applied on top and swiftly removed.

16. The working temperature of warm wax is approximately 43°C.

17. The growing hair is nourished via the dermal papilla.

18. The telogen stage in the hair growth cycle is the resting stage.

19. The changing stage of the hair growth cycle is called anagen.

20. Depilatory creams can irritate the skin if used too often.

21. Ingrowing hairs can occur if the area is not exfoliated regularly.

22. Ingrowing hairs only occur in people with strong hair growth.

23. The active ingredient in bleaching products is hydrogen peroxide.

24. After-wax lotion is mainly applied after waxing to remove any excess wax.

25. A skin test should be applied prior to *every* waxing treatment.

FINAL END TEST **ANSWERS**

1.	No	This is incorrect. It would be a definite contra-indication.
2.	Yes	
3.	Yes	
4.	Yes	This is a delicate area. Hot wax opens the follicle, and a skilled therapist who has had a lot of practice can make this treatment quite painless.
5.	Yes	
6.	Yes	
7.	Yes	
8.	No	Not so. Because of its higher working temperature, it can cause a heat reaction.
9.	Yes	
10.	Yes	
11.	No	Sugar paste is water-soluble and so is very easy to remove from the skin and heating units.
12.	Yes	
13.	Yes	
14.	Yes	

15. Yes
16. Yes
17. Yes
18. Yes
19. No   Anagen is the growing stage. The changing stage is catagen.
20. Yes
21. Yes
22. No   Ingrown hairs can occur on any type of hair growth. They are very common with a stronger hair growth.
23. Yes
24. No   After-wax lotion/oil is applied to soothe the area and reduce redness.
25. No   This is unnecessary. A sensitive skin, new client to waxing or a client with a history of sensitivity should have a skin test.

Marking Guide and Grading

Check your answers and then check them against the guide below. In percentage terms 60% is considered a pass. With this type of end test, because it's a simple Yes or No answer, there is a strong likelihood you could have guessed some of the answers! You should take this into account when determining your grade.

15 correct answers   a pass – well done

20 correct answers   a credit – excellent

Above 22 correct answers   is exceptional!
Below 15 correct answers means you need to spend more time revising, so go back to your course notes and Revision Maps, and then have another go.

CHAPTER EIGHT

TEAMWORK AND WORKING RELATIONS

CHECKLIST ✓ Can You?

	Yes	No	Page No
1. Discuss the importance of teamwork.			322
2. Outline methods of maintaining customer relations.			323
3. State what should be included in a job description.			324
4. Discuss the importance of appraisal and training, and the benefits of having long- and short-term targets.			325
5. Review some multiple choice and short answer questions around chapter content.			326
6. Answer questions around possible scenarios based on teamwork and working relations.			332
7. Attempt a final end test.			336

Normally in external examinations and end tests, questions around teamwork and working relations are infrequent. This is because this area is assessed in the salon situation, where your abilities in these areas can be more realistically judged.

However, some short answer and multiple choice questions are included for you to focus your revision and hopefully improve your practical performance. The chapter starts off with Revision Maps around the key factors of teamwork and working relations, and finishes with a short end test.

Revision Map – The Importance of Teamwork

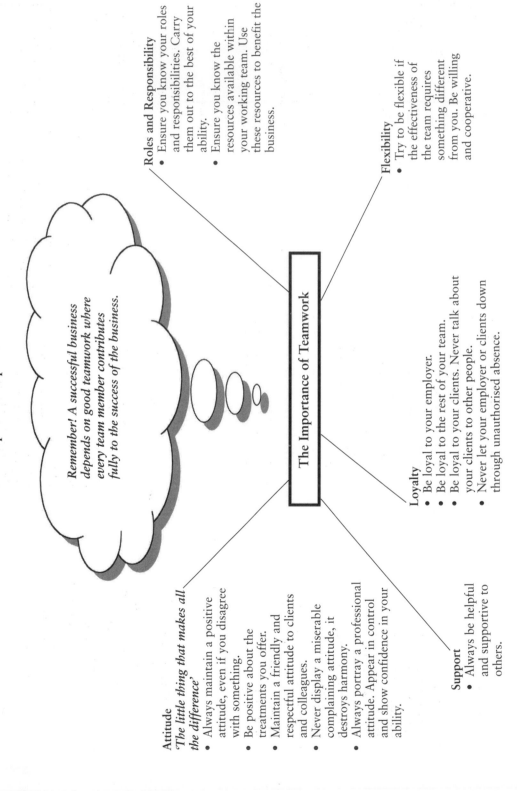

Remember! A successful business depends on good teamwork where every team member contributes fully to the success of the business.

The Importance of Teamwork

Roles and Responsibility
- Ensure you know your roles and responsibilities. Carry them out to the best of your ability.
- Ensure you know the resources available within your working team. Use these resources to benefit the business.

Flexibility
- Try to be flexible if the effectiveness of the team requires something different from you. Be willing and cooperative.

Loyalty
- Be loyal to your employer.
- Be loyal to the rest of your team.
- Be loyal to your clients. Never talk about your clients to other people.
- Never let your employer or clients down through unauthorised absence.

Attitude
'The little thing that makes all the difference'
- Always maintain a positive attitude, even if you disagree with something.
- Be positive about the treatments you offer.
- Maintain a friendly and respectful attitude to clients and colleagues.
- Never display a miserable complaining attitude, it destroys harmony.
- Always portray a professional attitude. Appear in control and show confidence in your ability.

Support
- Always be helpful and supportive to others.

Revision Map – Maintaining Customer Relations

Remember! Good manners cost nothing and can generate a lot of business.

Maintaining Customer Relations

Communication
- Be courteous; always check the customer understands what you are saying.
- Be sympathetic to individual's needs when dealing with overseas visitors or people with disabilities.
- Write clearly and spell the customer's name correctly.
- Do not use scruffy stationery.

Always project the desired image
- Wear salon uniform.
- Tidy hair, light make-up.
- Minimum jewellery.
- Be courteous and helpful.
- No negative behaviour.
- Ensure you know any rules and procedures you must comply with.

Try to meet the customers' needs by:
- Providing excellent treatments at all times.
- Dealing with complaints constructively.
- Seeking clarification or assistance from others if you need to.
- Being flexible, eg covering for absent colleagues.
- Explaining any limitations or problems honestly, eg if an item of equipment was suddenly broken and unable to be used.

Be responsible to customers' feelings
- Try to assess if the customer is nervous, anxious or annoyed.
- Give the customer an opportunity to convey their feelings.
- Treat complaints sensitively and in line with organisational procedures.
- Respond appropriately – eg calmly, apologetically, firmly.

Data Protection
- Never leave customer record cards lying around, to be read by others.
- Adhere to the Data Protection Act 1984 if you use a computer to keep records.

When dealing with complaints, make sure you know about the Sale of Goods Act 1994 and the Trade Descriptions Act 1968 and 1972.

Revision Map – Job Descriptions

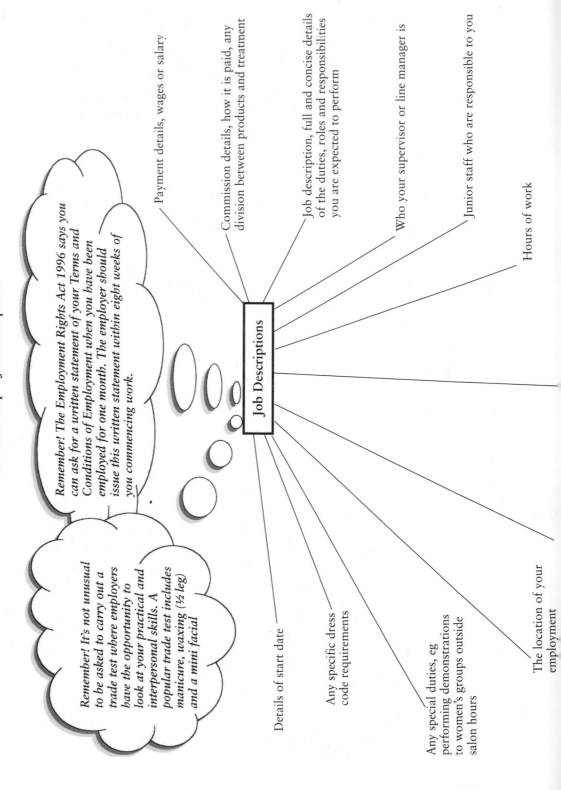

Remember! The Employment Rights Act 1996 says you can ask for a written statement of your Terms and Conditions of Employment when you have been employed for one month. The employer should issue this written statement within eight weeks of you commencing work.

Remember! It's not unusual to be asked to carry out a trade test where employers have the opportunity to look at your practical and interpersonal skills. A popular trade test includes manicure, waxing (½ leg) and a mini facial

Job Descriptions

Payment details, wages or salary

Commission details, how it is paid, any division between products and treatment

Job description, full and concise details of the duties, roles and responsibilities you are expected to perform

Who your supervisor or line manager is

Junior staff who are responsible to you

Hours of work

The location of your employment

Any special duties, eg performing demonstrations to women's groups outside salon hours

Any specific dress code requirements

Details of start date

Revision Map – Setting Targets in your Employment

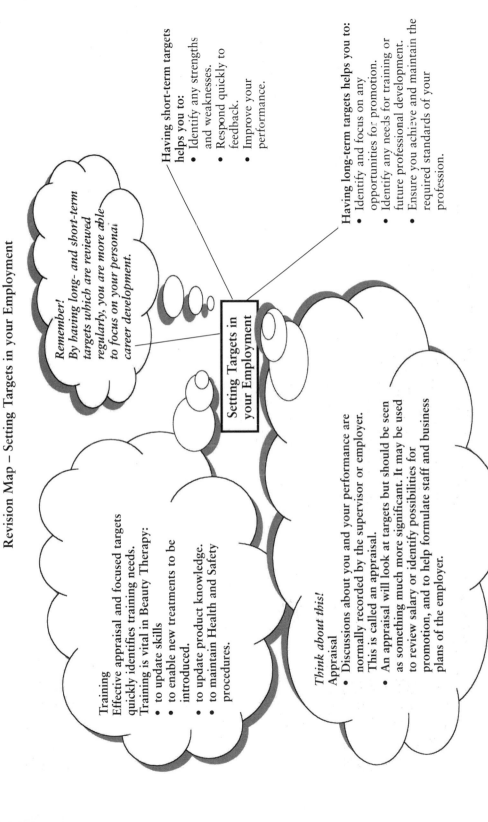

Setting Targets in your Employment

Remember!
By having long- and short-term targets which are reviewed regularly, you are more able to focus on your personal career development.

Having short-term targets helps you to:
- Identify any strengths and weaknesses.
- Respond quickly to feedback.
- Improve your performance.

Having long-term targets helps you to:
- Identify and focus on any opportunities for promotion.
- Identify any needs for training or future professional development.
- Ensure you achieve and maintain the required standards of your profession.

Training
Effective appraisal and focused targets quickly identifies training needs.
Training is vital in Beauty Therapy:
- to update skills
- to enable new treatments to be introduced.
- to update product knowledge.
- to maintain Health and Safety procedures.

Think about this!
Appraisal
- Discussions about you and your performance are normally recorded by the supervisor or employer. This is called an appraisal.
- An appraisal will look at targets but should be seen as something much more significant. It may be used to review salary or identify possibilities for promotion, and to help formulate staff and business plans of the employer.

SHORT ANSWER QUESTIONS

Q1. Why must the beauty therapist demonstrate a respectful approach at all times? *(4 marks)*

Answer: A respectful professional approach will encourage client confidence and loyalty, and will contribute to a harmonious salon environment for customers and staff members.

Q2. What are the advantages of wearing make-up in the working environment? *(2 marks)*

Answer: A well applied make-up application can portray a professional image and provide a pleasing example to clients.

Q3. How can the individual therapist project the image of the establishment that employs them? *(3 marks)*

Answer: The therapist can achieve this by:
• Always wearing a clean, pressed salon uniform.
• Ensuring they know of the establishment rules and procedures and complying with them at all times.
• Always behaving in a courteous and helpful manner.
• Using establishment resources as appropriate, eg:
  1 salon stationery/literature
  2 salon equipment
  3 salon consumables.

Q4. Why must beauty therapists be flexible in their approach to their job? *(5 marks)*

Answer: Flexibility is very important in any job that involves customer service. In beauty therapy establishments customers often arrive late for appointments, they sometimes change their mind about the treatment they have booked, and even send a friend or relative if they can't attend themselves. These occurrences must be met by a smiling therapist who is flexible and adaptable enough to adjust treatment times if appropriate, provide something entirely different if requested, and generally meet the individual needs of the client to the best of their abilities.

Q5. Briefly outline the Data Protection Act 1996. *(2 marks)*

Answer: This Act requires that any personal data *held on computer* is protected. Businesses using computers to store client information must register with the data protection registrar and comply with a code of practice.

Q6. Which Act stresses that goods must be 'fit for their purpose and as described'? *(1 mark)*

Answer: Sale and Supply of Goods Act 1994.

Q7. State three benefits of effective teamwork. *(6 marks)*

Answer:
• There is a more harmonious working environment.
• Everyone's individual and specialist skills are recognised, which contribute to individual job satisfaction and better use of staff resources for the employer.
• There is a better support network for all staff, especially new and junior staff.

Q8. Why does a job description contain details of a person's supervisor or line manager? *(1 mark)*

Answer: This person is named so that the new employee knows who they report to.

Q9. Outline four duties that a supervisor may have to undertake in the supervisory role of a new beauty therapist. *(4 marks)*

Answer:
• Welcome the new employee.
• Introduce the new employee to other team/staff members.
• Provide vital information, even training, to the new employee regarding the establishments procedures, eg till techniques, complaint procedures.
• Act as a mentor or person that the new employee can contact in the event of any queries or problems.
• Monitor the therapist's progress.
• Set short- and long-term targets for the therapist.

Q10. Can junior therapists ask for written details of their terms and conditions of employment? *(2 marks)*

Answer: Yes, an employee at any level can ask for a written statement of their terms and conditions of employment, under the Employment Rights Act 1996.

Q11. Why is it important to regularly identify any training needs an individual may have? *(4 marks)*

Answer: Because beauty therapy is a fast moving industry, new treatments and products are constantly being developed and marketed. The therapist must continually update their knowledge and skills to offer the best services to customers and maintain employability.

Q12. Explain briefly the differences between an appraisal and a review of targets? *(4 marks)*

Answer: In industry, appraisal is much more in depth than a review of targets, although a review of targets will be included in the appraisal process. An appraisal is a formal procedure which looks at an individual employee and their performance. It also tends to take place less frequently, eg annually.

Q13. What are the physical indications that are commonly displayed by a customer who is angry? *(4 marks)*

Answer: The body language is often aggressive, eg:
- The body held stiffly and positioned too closely to the other person.
- Excessive use of the arms or hands.
- Raised tone of voice, even shouting. Tone aggressive and sharp.
- Altered physical appearance, eg red face or neck.
- The client may be emotional or tearful.

Q14. Why should complaining clients be taken to a quieter area of the salon? *(3 marks)*

Answer: Because there is more chance of calming the client down in a quieter, calmer place. Also by dealing with the client away from other clients, any possible damage to the business is minimised.

Q15. How should the therapist alter their verbal communication when speaking to a client who speaks very little English?

Answer:

- Speak slowly and use simple words and statements.
- Check with the client that they have understood what has been said.
- Use visual aids or prompts if available.
- Try to focus their communication around what the client needs to know without unnecessary elaboration.

MULTIPLE CHOICE QUESTIONS

Some examples of multiple choice examination questions are included for you to enable you to give yourself a short test. Carefully consider the descriptions provided before choosing your answer. Only one answer is correct.
Indicate your answer by putting an **X** in the circle: ◯

Q1. What is a trade test?

a) a practical test carried out in college before a final assessment ◯

b) a practical test set by a prospective employer ◯

c) a practical test set by the awarding body ◯

d) a practical test designed by leading cosmetic manufacturers ◯

Q2. In what year did the Employment Rights Act become legislation?

a) 1964 ◯

b) 1968 ◯

c) 1992 ◯

d) 1996 ◯

Q3. Which one of the following is *not* normally included in a job description?

a) holiday entitlement ◯

b) hours of work ◯

c) the salon's gross profit figure ◯

d) details of notice required by the employer ◯

Q4. When dealing with a customer complaint regarding faulty goods, the therapist should:

a) follow establishment procedures ○

b) offer a credit note refund ○

c) offer a cash refund ○

d) refer the complaint to the receptionist ○

Q5. Why is nail enamel *not* worn by the beauty therapist during a facial treatment?

a) because it is a hygiene requirement ○

b) because only manicurists are allowed to wear enamel ○

c) because it can chip and look unattractive ○

d) because it may not match the salon uniform ○

Q6. If client record cards are stored solely in a central records box, the therapist should explain that:

a) all information given and recorded is protected by the Data Protection Act 1996 ○

b) all information given and recorded is not confidential and could be accessed by other staff members ○

c) all information given and recorded is confidential ○

d) all information given and recorded is not confidential because it is monitored under the Data Protection Act 1996 ○

Q7. What action should be taken if a client arrives ten minutes late for a 30 minute manicure treatment, during a fully booked Saturday session?

a) the client should be told to re-book the appointment ○

b) the therapist should refuse to carry out the treatment ○

c) the therapist should explain that a part treatment only can be carried out and the treatment begun immediately ○

d) the client should be charged a cancellation fee and offered a light beverage ○

Q8. If a client has booked for a facial steam and exfoliation treatment, and the facial steamer is broken, an appropriate action to be taken is to:

a) telephone the client and cancel the appointment ○

b) telephone the client and reschedule the appointment for a time when the steamer has been repaired ○

c) explain to the client on arrival what has happened and offer to perform a facial massage ○

d) explain to the client on arrival what has happened and advise her that you intend to use hot steam towels as an alternative to the facial steamer ○

Q9. Which one of the following can *damage* a harmonious working environment?

a) unreliability ○

b) loyalty ○

c) flexibility ○

d) consideration for others ○

Q10. Why should details of clients' complaints be recorded?

a) to blacklist clients who complain all the time ○

b) to enable the salon owner to determine how much time is spent dealing with complaints ○

c) as a prevention against damages claims ○

d) to allow the salon to monitor and act on complaints so improvements can be made ○

MULTIPLE CHOICE TEST – ANSWERS

1.	B		6.	B
2.	D		7.	C
3.	C		8.	D
4.	A		9.	A
5.	A		10.	D

Marking and Grading

8 correct   a credit, excellent

6 correct   a pass, well done

Below 4   you need to spend more time revising. Look again at your
course notes and the Revision Maps, and have another go in a
week's time

SCENARIOS

Sometimes examples of situations or scenarios are presented to the student,
and questions are asked about the best way to act to bring about a solution.
Obviously these type of questions are popular if an assessor needs to test a
student in an area that has not been observed, eg dealing with a client
complaint. Students should always ensure they know *establishment procedures*
for dealing with complaints. Students should also ensure they know any
establishment policies and rules and should adhere to them as far as possible.

Some examples of possible scenarios follow, accompanied by some sample
questions and answers. Reviewing the scenarios will help to focus your revision
and provide some common sense guidelines in this personal, difficult, yet
important, area.

Scenario One

The salon has appointed a new receptionist. The receptionist is having some
problems in the scheduling of appointments. On two occasions you have been
double-booked with clients, you have missed your lunch break once, and have
had to stay late on your afternoon off due to a booking error.

You arrive at work and see that you are solidly booked all day and no time has
been allowed in between clients to tidy up and set up for the next treatment.
Furthermore, the receptionist has booked a manicure client through your lunch
break.

Q1. What action should be taken?

Answer:
• Avoid any kind of verbal attack on the receptionist, because quite clearly they are in need of some serious staff training.
• Approach the supervisor and explain the position clearly and calmly.
• Ask if it would be possible to reassign the manicure client to another therapist.
• Closely review the bookings to see if it is necessary to reassign any other clients, or if realistically you can get through the day without clients waiting or their receiving an inferior service.
• Ask if the junior/trainee therapist can assist you during changeover and preparation.
• Accept some blame for this situation occurring, because you have not highlighted the difficulties you have previously experienced.

Q2. What should be included in a training programme for the receptionist?

Answer: From the information provided, the receptionist needs training in the scheduling of appointments.
• Training should be given in acceptable time allocations for treatments which should include a *short period* of tidying-up time.
• Any particular salon policies regarding preparation must be discussed with the receptionist; eg if the therapist remains 15 minutes after the last client of the day to prepare for the next day and clean and sterilise equipment, or if the therapist commences work 15 minutes prior to the first appointment for preparation.
• An observation session may be included when the receptionist shadows a therapist performing minor less personal treatments, thus enabling the receptionist to gain an insight into what exactly is involved.

Scenario Two
During a pedicure treatment, the client begins to tell you of her dissatisfaction with the quality of service she has received during a lash tinting treatment with another therapist.

Q1. What action should be taken by the therapist?

Answer: In this unpleasant situation, the therapist should tactfully and respectfully explain that they are unable to comment but on completion of the pedicure treatment the supervisor will be sought and the discussion can be continued with that person.

Q2. What action should be taken by the supervisior?

Answer: The supervisor should follow establishment procedures for dealing with complaints. This will normally involve some or all of the following:
- Allowing the client to explain why they are dissatisfied.
- Listening without interrupting.
- Clarifying any points that are unclear.
- Making a judgement, does the client have a genuine complaint or not?
- Negotiating an acceptable solution and carrying the solution out.
- Remaining calm and polite throughout.
- Recording details of the complaint as appropriate.
- Discussing the complaint with the employee involved.
- Implementing training for the employee if deemed to be required.
- Demonstrating sensitivity to both the customer's and employee's feelings throughout.

Scenario Three

Look at the sample appointment page for a morning session.
Consider the following information:

- *Paul is the only therapist qualified to offer sculptured nail treatments.*
- *Cathy is the epilation specialist, but all other therapists can safely and competently carry out epilation.*
- *The electric foot spa is discovered to be faulty.*

Paul telephones Mary at 8.45 am and informs her that his car will not start. He is rushing to catch a train which will get him to work for 9.45 am.

Q1. What action can be taken to ensure Mr Holmes undergoes his treatment?

Answer: Mary is the only person free who could take over Mr Holmes' treatment. However, this would require cancellation of the meeting with Gala Cosmetics at extremely short notice. Alternatively, Gala Cosmetics could be asked to reschedule a meeting for later in the day if convenient.

Q2. The electric foot spa is broken. To whom should this be reported, and how should the equipment be dealt with?

Answer: Mary should be informed about the broken equipment, and it should be taken out of service immediately. All staff should be told of the unavailability of this piece of equipment.

FRIDAY NOVEMBER 5TH			
	CATHY	SUSAN	MARY (MANAGERESS)	PAUL
9.00	June Jones Epilation	J Hammond Facial/Manicure	Meeting with cosmetic rep from 'GALA'	Mr Holmes Gentlemen's facial with steam
9.15		Pedicure/Footspa		
9.30	Miss Ryan Cleanse & Make-up			
10.00				Mrs Smith Sculptured nails (incomplete set)
10.15	Heather Mills Epilation			
10.30	K Singh Manicure			
10.45				
11.00		K Smyth	C Morgan Specialist facial with steam	
11.15	R Moore Epilation			
11.30				Mrs Bouquet consultation/advice
11.45	B Needwel Epilation	C Hoover Eyebrow shape		
12.00	Afternoon off		Mrs Milani Waxing full leg U/A, B/L	John Hanks Back massage
12.15		LUNCH		
12.30				LUNCH
12.45				
13.00				
13.15			LUNCH	
13.30				

Q3. Cathy informs Mary that she would like to leave at 11.30 because she has a serious problem at her son's school, and the headmistress has offered her a 12.00 appointment. Who could carry out the 11.45 a.m. appointment for Mrs B Needwel?

Answer: Paul is the only person free to carry out the treatment on Mrs Needwel.

Q4. Identify any staff training needs that this team of therapists may have.

Answer: The female team members need training in sculptured nail techniques.

Q5. What details are normally required when making appointments? Are any important details omitted from the example appointment sheet?

Answer:
- The client's name, the treatment required and a contact telephone number should be recorded when making appointments.
- No contact numbers were available for any of the clients listed in the example.
- No name was entered for the representative from the cosmetics company.
- The requirements of K Smyth booked with Susan were not recorded.

FINAL END TEST

This section consists of statements. Each one may be correct or incorrect. The answer required is simply

> Yes or No.

In your assessment of whether the statement is correct or incorrect, you must only base your answer on the information provided.

1. Employers are obliged to give you the holiday weeks of your choice.

2. A negative attitude to work restricts a persons promotion opportunities.

3. Being flexible at work allows senior staff to exploit junior staff.

4. Clients can pick up an unhappy working atmosphere.

5. The Data Protection Act 1996 refers to records kept on computer.

6. If a customer has a hearing loss and lip reads what is said, the therapist should aim to speak clearly and look directly at the customer.

7. An effective team recognises an individual's contribution.

8. Out-of-date salon price lists should be disposed of.

9. If a therapist is unsure of something, they should seek assistance and clarification from others.

10. The therapist should endeavour to wear the salon uniform at all times.

11. A job description should include details of hours of work, payment and the salon's weekly takings.

12. Asking an individual to undergo a trade test is against the law.

13. An appraisal can be used to focus the employee on their performance and aspirations.

14. Following an appraisal, it is normal that both the appraiser and the employee sign any documentation used or agreed in the appraisal.

⬭

15. Ongoing training and updating is very important to a successful career in beauty therapy.

⬭

16. It is unacceptable to discuss clients and fellow colleagues with others.

⬭

17. Sometimes it is necessary to cancel and reschedule appointments.

⬭

18. Being loyal to your employer helps build a happy working environment.

⬭

19. Negative body language from the therapist can be off-putting to clients and make the client feel ill at ease.

⬭

20. Establishment policies and procedures can be overruled if the therapist prefers.

⬭

FINAL END TEST **ANSWERS**

1. No   Holidays are negotiable.
2. Yes   Quite true, employers are unlikely to promote a negative employee.
3. No   All staff members need to be flexible and work as a team. Exploitation must be stamped out immediately.
4. Yes
5. Yes
6. Yes
7. Yes
8. Yes
9. Yes

10. Yes
11. No   Salon takings would not be included in a job description.
12. No   Untrue; it is common practice in beauty therapy.
13. Yes
14. Yes
15. Yes
16. Yes
17. Yes
18. Yes
19. Yes
20. No   Establishment policies and procedures should never be overruled. This behaviour could lead to disciplinary action from the employer.

Marking Guide and Grading

The marking guide is provided to help and encourage you to monitor your progress. This style of end test has been chosen to reinforce some key revision points, to further assist your revision process. Obviously, if you have guessed a lot of the answers, it will not give you a proper reflection of the true grade you have achieved, and really, if you have guessed answers, you need to revise a bit more.

17 correct   a credit

15 correct   a confident pass

13 correct   a borderline pass

Below 10 means you need to revise a bit more. Go back to your course notes and Revision Maps, spend some more time studying, and have another go at the test at a later date. Don't be put off, but be prepared to spend some proper time on it.

FINAL MULTIPLE CHOICE END TEST

The end test entails 80 questions devised around the different areas covered in the text, except for Chapter 8.

You should allow yourself two hours if you wish to complete the test in one sitting. If you prefer to tackle the test in smaller segments, a good rule of thumb is to allow 30 minutes to answer 20 questions.

The spread of questions or test specification for this test is as follows:-

Topic	Percentage
1. Product knowledge	24%
2. Beauty therapy processes	24%
3. Health and safety	16%
4. Anatomy	21%
5. Contra-indications	15%

Carefully consider the alternatives provided before choosing your answer. Only one answer is correct. Indicate your answer by putting an **X** in the circle: ◯

Q1. **Why should a freshly laundered overall be worn daily?**

a) it is a rule under COSHH regulations   ◯

b) it helps maintain hygiene standards   ◯

c) it looks nice   ◯

d) it is a requirement of local bye-laws   ◯

Q2. **Which fire extinguisher can be used on a burning wax pot?**

a) yellow – foam   ◯

b) red – water   ◯

c) black – carbon dioxide   ◯

d) a light duty fire blanket   ◯

Q3. **The nail bed has:**

a) no corrugations   ◯

b) a reduced blood supply   ◯

c) a rich blood supply   ◯

d) an absence of lymphatic ducts   ◯

Q4. Which one of the following statements is correct? Paronychia is:

a) a viral infection ○

b) an infection which affects the tissues around the nail plate ○

c) non-contagious ○

d) a condition which is contagious and affects the nail plate ○

Q5. What are transverse lines across the nail plate commonly called?

a) beau's lines ○

b) onychorrhexis ○

c) onychomycosis ○

d) leukonychia ○

Q6. Which one of the following is the reproducing area of the nail?

a) eponychium ○

b) nail bed ○

c) matrix ○

d) lunula ○

Q7. What is the active ingredient in cuticle milk?

a) potassium hydroxide ○

b) hydrogen peroxide ○

c) lanolin ○

d) gum tragacanth ○

Q8. What is cuticle oil used for?

a) strengthen the cuticles ○

b) prevent the nail from drying out ○

c) dry the nail enamel application ○

d) remove excess cuticle ○

Q9. Acetone is best described as a:

a) byproduct of soap manufacture ○

b) colourant ○

c) nourisher ○

d) solvent ○

Q10. Which one of the following is a contra-indication to a pedicure treatment?

a) corns ○

b) a bunion ○

c) pterygium ○

d) onychia ○

Q11. A cuticle knife is used to:

a) remove excess cuticle stuck to the nail plate ○

b) ease back the cuticles ○

c) clean under the free edge of the nail ○

d) remove hangnails ○

Q12. Which *one* of the following is a contra-indication to facial massage?

a) a client suffering with a headache ○

b) heart conditions ○

c) a dry sensitive skin type ○

d) a client with sensitive eyes ○

Q13. The glass bead steriliser is used for sterilising:

a) Make-up brushes ○

b) tweezers ○

c) plastic items ○

d) spatulas ○

Q14. What is the time required to complete the sterilisation process in an autoclave at 121°C?

a) 5 minutes ○

b) 10 minutes ○

c) 15 minutes ○

d) 20 minutes ○

Q15. An example of a chemical sterilising agent is?

a) witch-hazel ◯

b) an antiseptic ◯

c) liquid soap ◯

d) bleach ◯

Q16. The 'S' in the abbreviation COSHH stands for:

a) sterilisation ◯

b) solvents ◯

c) solutions ◯

d) substances ◯

Q17. Which Act requires ear-piercers and electrologists to register with the local authority?

a) the Environmental Protection Act 1990 ◯

b) the Health and Safety at Work Act 1974 ◯

c) the Local Government (Miscellaneous Provisions) Act 1982 ◯

d) the Management of Health and Safety at Work Regulations 1992 ◯

Q18. Eyelash tint comes under COSHH Regulations because it is:

a) caustic ◯

b) sensitising ◯

c) irritant ◯

d) flammable ◯

Q19. Which one of the following are the most resistant micro-organisms?

a) fungi ◯

b) germs ◯

c) bacterium ◯

d) viruses ◯

Q20. Who is responsible for assessing the risks in the manual handling of stock?

a) the employee ○

b) the employer ○

c) the technician ○

d) the person delivering the stock ○

Q21. Which *one* of the following would contra-indicate an ozone vapour, facial steaming treatment?

a) Milia ○

b) Migraine sufferers ○

c) bronchial conditions ○

d) acne vulgaris ○

Q22. Skin cleansing is performed prior to mask therapy in order to:

a) Moisturise the skin ○

b) desquamate the skin ○

c) free the skin of surface secretions and make-up ○

d) produce an erythema ○

Q23. Which one of the following is the *best* choice of cleanser and toner for a dry skin?

a) cleansing lotion and orangeflower water ○

b) cleansing cream and rosewater ○

c) cleansing emulsion and orangeflower water ○

d) cleansing cream and witch-hazel ○

Q24. Which *one* of the following statements is correct?

a) a night treatment cream should only be used on dry mature skin ○

b) a night treatment cream is suitable for use on the face, neck and eyes ○

c) a night treatment cream is for the over-forties age group only ○

d) a night treatment cream can be used to improve dry skin conditions ○

Q25. Which one of the following best describes a mature skin?

a) small pores, dry flaky appearance ◯

b) small pores, poor colour and texture, deep lines and wrinkles, even crepeyness ◯

c) poor colour and texture, lines around the eyes and forehead ◯

d) broken veins on the cheeks, lines around the eyes and neck ◯

Q26. Brush cleansing treatments are used to:

a) deep cleanse and exfoliate the skin ◯

b) remove lines and wrinkles ◯

c) reduce a florid complexion ◯

d) cure acne conditions ◯

Q27. A pH balanced cleansing bar for the skin will have a pH balance of:

a) 1–2 ◯

b) 4.5–5.5 ◯

c) 7 ◯

d) 9.5–10.5 ◯

Q28. Which one of the following is *least* suitable for an oily skin type as a toning product?

a) witch-hazel ◯

b) astringent ◯

c) orangeflower water ◯

d) rosewater ◯

Q29. A contra-indication which would prevent a facial treatment being carried out is:

a) vitiligo ◯

b) sensitive skin ◯

c) lentigo ◯

d) impetigo ◯

Q30. Vapour steaming is used in facial treatments in order to?

a) slow down the growth of bacteria on the skin ○

b) open the pores, desquamate the skin, soften the stratum germinitivum ○

c) increase circulation, open the pores and soften stratum corneum ○

d) relax nervous clients ○

Q31. Which one of the following is a suitable eyelash tinting colour for an elderly client with white hair and blue eyes?

a) grey ○

b) blue/black ○

c) black ○

d) brown/black ○

Q32. What strength of hydrogen peroxide should be used in an eyelash tinting treatment?

a) 5 vol ○

b) 10 vol ○

c) 15 vol ○

d) 20 vol ○

Q33. The lasting effect of a lash and brow tinting treatment is:

a) 1 week ○

b) 2 weeks ○

c) 4–6 weeks ○

d) 2 months ○

Q34. Individual false eyelashes can stay in place for up to:

a) 1 week ○

b) 2 weeks ○

c) 4 weeks ○

d) 6 weeks ○

Q35. Why is a patch test carried out prior to the application of false eyelashes?

a) to see if the client is allergic to the eyelashes

b) to see is the client is allergic to the adhesive

c) to see if the client is allergic to eye cosmetics

d) because it looks professional

Q36. Which one of the following is a suitable eyelash tinting colour for a young client with blue eyes and blond hair, who wants a fun summery look?

a) brown

b) grey

c) blue/black

d) black/brown

Q37. Eyelash tinting treatments are carried out with the client in a semi-reclining position because:

a) it makes application and removal easier for the therapist

b) it is a requirement under health and safety procedures

c) it is a requirement of local bye-laws

d) it is a requirement of COSHH regulations

Q38. Where is the occiptal bone found?

a) at the front of the head

b) at the back of the head

c) at the side of the head

d) at the top of the head

Q39. Which bones are found above and around the ear?

a) temporal bones

b) parietal bones

c) mandible

d) zygomatic bones

Q40. Which bones carry the upper teeth?

a) mandible ○

b) zygomatic bones ○

c) maxillae ○

d) scapula ○

Q41. What is the thinner bone of the forearm?

a) radius ○

b) ulna ○

c) tibia ○

d) carpus ○

Q42. Which *one* of the following would contra-indicate an eyebrow shaping treatment?

a) conjunctivitis ○

b) a slight headache ○

c) the client has just undergone an eyebrow tint ○

d) a cold sore on the upper lip ○

Q43. Automatic tweezers are more appropriate for use on clients with:

a) a high pain threshold ○

b) fine eyebrow hair ○

c) a low pain threshold ○

d) scar tissue in the eyebrows ○

Q44. Which *one* of the following would contra-indicate an eyelash and eyebrow tint?

a) if a patch test was negative ○

b) if a patch test had not been carried out ○

c) a skin tag on the eyelid ○

d) if the client wears contact lenses ○

Q45. Clients with protruding eyes should be advised to use:

a) light coloured, frosty eyeshadows ○

b) darker matt eye colours and a touch of highlighter ○

c) matt light eyeshadow on the inner corners of the eye and dark matt colours on the outer corners ○

d) a dark lash building mascara instead of eyeshadow ○

Q46. A long face shape can be improved by:

a) shading the top of the forehead and chin ○

b) shading the lower jaw and cheekbones ○

c) highlighting the top of the forehead and chin ○

d) highlighting the side edges of the face ○

Q47. A suitable lip colour choice to wear with a deep mauve suit would be:

a) a shade of peach ○

b) a shade of beige or brown ○

c) a shade of pink ○

d) a neutral gloss ○

Q48. Why is a bridal make-up package charged differently to a special occasion make-up treatment?

a) clients are willing to pay more for this service because it is their wedding day ○

b) this service requires additional make-up products to be purchased by the salon. ○

c) this service generally involves a rehearsal and extra planning ○

d) on the day, extra time is to be allocated to the bride to make allowance for nerves ○

Q49. Colour correction is normally carried out in the make-up sequence:

a) by negotiation with the client ○

b) by carefully choosing the colour of face powder ○

c) at the end by balancing colours ○

d) at the moisturising stage ○

Q50. A cream foundation is more suitable for:

a) an oily skin ○

b) a dry skin ○

c) an acne skin ○

d) a client who requires a natural coverage ○

Q51. Magnesium carbonate is a common ingredient in:

a) mascara ○

b) foundation ○

c) face powder ○

d) lipstick ○

Q52. Frosting or iridescence in cosmetic products can be produced by the addition of:

a) mica ○

b) zinc oxide ○

c) magnesium stearate ○

d) beeswax ○

Q53. The tough fibrous layer of the dermis is the:

a) subcutis ○

b) papillary layer ○

c) germinating layer ○

d) reticular layer ○

Q54. The arrector pili muscle is found in the:

a) epidermis ○

b) dermis ○

c) sebaceous gland ○

d) subcutis ○

Q55. The secretion from the sudoriferous glands, is commonly called:

a) sweat

b) sebum

c) water

d) tissue fluid

Q56. Which *one* of the following occurs when the body is too hot?

a) vaso constriction

b) contraction of the arrector pili muscle

c) vaso dilation

d) reduced activity from the sudoriferous glands

Q57. Which one of the following muscles is found in the eyebrow region?

a) orbicularis oris

b) procerus

c) lavator labii

d) triangularis

Q58. Which *one* of the following is a muscle of mastication?

a) platysma

b) corrugator

c) mentalis

d) temporalis

Q59. Which one of the following has a mild toning action when used in a facial mask combination?

a) china clay

b) orangeflower water

c) magnesium carbonate

d) witch-hazel

Q60. A massage routine for a client requiring a stimulating invigoration effect would include:

a) extra effleurage ◯

b) extra vibration and tapotement ◯

c) restricted petrissage ◯

d) restricted tapotement ◯

Q61. A suitable mask for a dry and very sensitive skin type is:

a) calamine and distilled water ◯

b) magnesium carbonate and orangeflower water ◯

c) magnesium carbonate and rosewater ◯

d) almond oil and kaolin ◯

Q62. A hot oil mask treatment is unsuitable for:

a) heavily lined skin ◯

b) mature skin ◯

c) dry skin ◯

d) florid skin ◯

Q63. Which one of the following statements best describes arteries?

a) arteries carry oxygenated blood; they have thick muscular walls ◯

b) arteries have muscular walls and carry oxygenated blood ◯

c) arteries lie deep in the tissues and contain valves ◯

d) arteries run alongside veins and have thin walls ◯

Q64. To comply with health and safety legislation, what action should the professional therapist take if he/she is unsure of how to carry out a cleansing treatment with the salon's mechanical brush cleansing equipment?

a) have a trial run with a colleague ◯

b) contact the manufacturer for an instruction book ◯

c) ask the supervisor for training ◯

d) omit brush cleansing from any treatments given ◯

Q65. Which legislation states that the employer should have fire extinguishers regularly serviced?

a) COSHH regulations

b) Electricity at Work Regulations 1990

c) Fire Precautions Act 1971

d) Provision and Use of Work Equipment Regulations 1992

Q66. Which *one* of the following areas is best treated with hot delipatory wax?

a) a dense, coarse bikini line

b) a fine, fair bikini line

c) medium coarse hair on the upper lip on a heat sensitive client

d) eyebrow hair

Q67. The working temperature of cool wax is approximately:

a) 20°C

b) 35°C

c) 43°C

d) 60°C

Q68. Which one of the following conditions is termed a systemic disorder?

a) extensive scarring

b) moles

c) bruising

d) diabetes mellitus

Q69. Which one of the following is a stimulating, brisk, intermittent massage movement?

a) slapping

b) deep friction circles

c) palmer kneading

d) digital stroking

Q70. The normal reaction to a hot wax treatment is:

a) irritation that fades within one hour ○

b) swelling in the area ○

c) erythema ○

d) tenderness and soreness in the area ○

Q71. The hair is nourished in the hair follicle by the:

a) sebaceous gland ○

b) dermal papilla ○

c) papillary layer of the epidermis ○

d) papillary layer of the dermis ○

Q72. A resting hair follicle is said to be in:

a) catagen ○

b) anagen ○

c) early anagen ○

d) telogen ○

Q73. Which one of the following is a contra-indication to warm waxing of the lower legs?

a) moles ○

b) varicose veins ○

c) scar tissue ○

d) a dry skin condition with some ingrowing hairs ○

Q74. Why is an antiseptic after-wax product applied following waxing?

a) to close the pores ○

b) to remove any traces of the waxing product which could come into contact with the client's clothes ○

c) to reduce the presence of micro-organisms on the skin, thus maintaining hygiene requirements ○

d) because the product has a lingering fragrance ○

Q75. Which one of the following would prevent a hair bleaching treatment going ahead?

a) a negative result to a patch test ◯

b) the presence of a thin, fine skin condition ◯

c) the presence of a dry skin condition ◯

d) the presence of sunburn in the area to be treated ◯

Q76. A completely natural depilatory product is:

a) sugaring paste ◯

b) warm wax ◯

c) hot wax ◯

d) hair removing cream ◯

Q77. The gastrocnemius is a muscle found:

a) at the front of the lower leg ◯

b) at the back of the lower leg ◯

c) in the lower forearm ◯

d) at the front of the body in the chest region ◯

Q78. The phalanges are the:

a) long bones of the hand ◯

b) bones of the ankle ◯

c) long bones of the feet ◯

d) bones that make up the fingers ◯

Q79. How frequently should an oily skin type use an exfoliation product?

a) weekly ◯

b) fortnightly ◯

c) every month ◯

d) every three months ◯

Q80. Which one of the following conditions is unsuitable for a facial massage treatment?

a) sensitive skin ⭕

b) pigmented skin ⭕

c) loose skin ⭕

d) a dry skin with a lot of milia ⭕

FINAL MULTIPLE CHOICE END TEST – ANSWERS

1.	B	21.	C	41.	B	61.	A
2.	C	22.	C	42.	A	62.	D
3.	C	23.	B	43.	C	63.	B
4.	B	24.	D	44.	B	64.	C
5.	A	25.	B	45.	B	65.	C
6.	C	26.	A	46.	A	66.	A
7.	A	27.	B	47.	C	67.	C
8.	B	28.	D	48.	C	68.	D
9.	D	29.	D	49.	D	69.	A
10.	D	30.	C	50.	B	70.	C
11.	A	31.	A	51.	C	71.	B
12.	B	32.	B	52.	A	72.	D
13.	B	33.	C	53.	D	73.	B
14.	C	34.	D	54.	B	74.	C
15.	D	35.	B	55.	A	75.	D
16.	D	36.	C	56.	C	76.	A
17.	C	37.	B	57.	B	77.	B
18.	B	38.	B	58.	D	78.	D
19.	D	39.	A	59.	C	79.	A
20.	B	40.	C	60.	B	80.	C

Marking and Grading

60 correct   a credit, excellent

48 correct   a pass, well done

Just below 45   you're nearly there. Keep revising, review the Revision Maps and have another go

Below 30   you need to spend more time revising. Look again at your course notes and the Revision Maps, and have another go in a week's time

BEAUTY THERAPY STUDY SKILLS